MAN UP
TO INFERTILITY

A personal and biblical journey through
infertility and adoption

PETE ROSCOE

malcolm down

PUBLISHING

First published 2020 by Malcolm Down Publishing Ltd.
www.malcolmdown.co.uk

24 23 22 21 20   7 6 5 4 3 2 1

British Library Cataloguing in Publication Data
A catalogue record for this book is available from the British Library.

ISBN 978-1-912863-34-1

Unless otherwise indicated, Scripture quotations taken from:

New International Version (Anglicised edition)
Copyright ©1979, 1984, 2011 by Biblica
(formerly International Bible Society).
Used by permission of Hodder & Stoughton Publishers,
an Hachette UK company.
All rights reserved.
'NIV' is a registered trademark of Biblica
(formerly International Bible Society).
UK trademark number 1448790.
Common English Bible
New Living Translation
King James Version
The author has added italics to Scripture quotations for emphasis.

Cover design by Esther Kotecha
Art direction by Sarah Grace

Printed in the UK

Contents

Acknowledgements

The first person I want to thank is my beautiful best friend and incredible wife Emma. She's been incredibly brave, constantly positive and pushes me to be better every day.

> 'He who finds a wife finds what is good and receives favour from the LORD.'
>
> *Proverbs 18 v 22*

To the three beautiful children we've been blessed with, you've completely turned our lives upside down but filled them with love and joy. This book is for all of you. We're praying you grow in wisdom, stature and favour with God and all the people you meet.

To all our friends and family who have been supporting and praying for us for so long thanks so much for your loyalty – it's meant so much to us and more than we can express.

Big thanks to Ems Hancock for giving me the push I needed to get this finished, to Richard P for help and advice with the book and to Malcolm Down for publishing and believing in this book.

I hope and pray this book's a blessing to you.

Pete

Foreword

Every day when I wake up, I look to the left of the bed and see photographs on the wall of people who are dear to us, that Zoe and I pray for every day. Many of these photos are couples dealing with issues of infertility. Every child is of course a miracle, but I am so grateful to God that over the years we have been able to add to some photos a birth date. But while some still wait, we pray on.

As my friend J.John puts it, 'we live between miracle and mystery.' This book is for those who know that betweenness very well, and will not only provide a great comfort but also guidance and very practical help from one who has navigated the journey personally.

In over 25 years of pastoral leadership (including Ivy, which Pete and his wife Emma were part of for many years), I have found many women courageously and openly able to talk about the vale of tears they have walked, or are walking as they wait. They may find others to share and care and be vulnerable with, and as the Bible puts it, they are even able to comfort others with the comfort they themselves have received.

Not so with the men.

Such subjects are not usually spoken about when we are growing up (and if they are, not well). The cultural and societal expectations on what makes a real man means the taboos remain and, for some, fester deep down as a hidden source of pain and even shame. Proverbs says, 'Hope deferred makes the heart sick,' and to stop that happening I was thrilled when my friend Dr Pete Roscoe wrote this book; it's a prescription for hope.

I read it straight through in one sitting and at the end shouted, 'Finally! Here is a book that is real about the problems yet also full of hope.' This is a sensitive and sensible book I can trust to put into the hands of men and their wives that is full of stories and truths that resonate. Through reading and discussing together, I believe they will grow closer together and to God, whether they are at the beginning of a time of questioning, going through a long-term process of prayer and decision-making about procedures, or coming to terms with all kinds of loss that we inevitably go through.

Read it, underline it, talk about it. My prayer is that God speaks to you through it as he did to me.

And if you picked this up wondering whether this is the book to help that man or couple you know, it is.

Rev Anthony Delaney
Leader, Ivy Church Network

Introduction

It has been a pretty humbling experience writing a book about overcoming infertility while we've still not yet had a birth child. You wouldn't read a book on golf by someone who can't play golf and neither would you pay a driving instructor to teach you to drive if they couldn't drive themselves. God likes to do things differently though. The Bible is littered with stories of underqualified men and women who God uses to fulfil his divine purposes. So, before I go on much further, I'll address the big white elephant in the room. I'm sorry if you think writing a book about overcoming infertility by a man struggling to overcome it himself is stupid – it probably is! I'll tell you a bit about myself. I'm just a normal everyday guy, I love my family, I'm most happy when I'm outdoors, and cycling and football are two of my big passions. I am a doctor but my speciality certainly isn't fertility medicine! What I'm getting at is that I'm not really qualified to be writing this book, I'm just being obedient to what God's called me to do, and that's all that He requires of us. People in Noah's generation would have thought it was 'absurd' for him to build the ark, it seemed 'crazy' for Naaman to take a dip in the dirty River Jordan, sheer 'recklessness' for David to fight a fully armoured giant with a sling and stone and 'madness' for God to entrust his only Son and mankind's eternal salvation to an unmarried teenager and an initially reluctant adoptive father. I'm certainly not comparing myself to these Bible heroes but when He asks us to do things that we and the world may regard as 'stupid or foolishness' we know that we are not the first people to tread this ground. If one man (or woman) is helped by the experiences that my wife and I have been through then all of this difficult time will have been worthwhile. As Paul says: '"My grace is sufficient for you, for my power is made perfect in weakness." Therefore I will boast all the more gladly about my weaknesses, so that Christ's power may rest on me.' (2 Corinthians 12:9)

My prayer for you as you read this book is not simply that you and your wife will have a family (I do pray for that as well!) but that you will find strength from the stories of modern-day men like you and me and the stories from the Bible of the men and women who faced this struggle and ultimately overcame. The men and women who still followed God even though it made no sense, did incredible acts and ended up changing history. I pray also that the stories in this book will help you to avoid years of bitterness and prevent you from living in the wilderness of disappointment and experience the true adventure that is living lives sold out for Jesus. That is why I'm writing this book – so men can live in freedom and oneness with our Father and God.

The longer I've been on this journey the more I have come to realise what overcoming looks like. Overcoming doesn't necessarily mean having a child. You could have a large family, but if your marriage is failing, your walk with God is non-existent and your life is bearing no fruit for the kingdom that's not an overcoming life.

Sadly, infertility is a very common problem which currently affects one in seven couples in the United Kingdom. If you aren't personally affected by it, no doubt you'll know someone who is maybe a friend, relative or even one of your own children. There are quite a lot of good Christian books available on journeying infertility which my wife has been reading, but a lot are aimed at women – what about us men? Women suffer with infertility in a different way to men. Women are often better able to share their pain with friends and family in ways that men often can't. Men often suffer in silence and find it incredibly hard to talk about. It's a taboo topic which can make us feel 'less manly'. One of my friends who has been on the journey too said he'd wished at the time that he could have just broken down and cried, but he couldn't. It's incredibly isolating. We feel like we've got to be strong for our wives but deep down the pain is real and it hurts. For my wife and I this has truly been the hardest time of our lives.

I felt God tell me to write this book after my wife Emma finally got pregnant but then had a miscarriage. I told God, 'There's no way I'm writing that now! No-one's going to be interested in reading a book about overcoming miscarriage and infertility unless the author has actually overcome it! That's stupid!'

A few months later, after some ministry time with a wise old pastor, I heard God speak to my heart again.

'Write that book.'

'Really?'

'Yes!'

'But it's still stupid!'

'I want you to write it.'

So here it is. This book is to help all the guys out there who are struggling in silence. The Petes who are supporting Emmas, the Zacks who are holding up Tamaras, guys like you and me struggling but want to overcome. My own testimony is the first part of the book and I've also asked some friends to share their own stories of overcoming infertility too.

Thankfully for us the Bible is also full of stories of great men and women who by the grace of God managed to triumph over their barrenness. In the second part of the book we'll study these stories from the husband's point of view and attempt to find ways we can learn from their strengths and weaknesses to help us better support our wives, grow closer to our Heavenly Father and ultimately overcome.

In the third and final part we will study how God has used adoption for some of the most significant men and women in the Bible and how God uses them in his ultimate plan to adopt everyone into his eternal family.

This book is specifically about the challenges of facing infertility, but you may be facing barrenness in a different area of your life, such as sickness, loss of faith or a loved one who is not yet saved. I believe the principles of this book will apply to those situations too.

This book tells stories of God's consistent love for mankind, hope triumphing over despair, love overcoming disappointment and joy being found where it wasn't expected. It's a journey for men who, with God's help, were able to 'man up' to infertility, partner with their wives and live overcoming lives.

If you've been encouraged by this book I'd love to hear about it! Please get in touch at manuptoinfertility@gmail.com

PART ONE

The Everyday Men

You are all going to have a different story but at the core I believe our struggles are often similar. I will share my personal story with you followed by the testimonies of some amazing guys I know who have kindly shared their journeys with you too so we can all learn more together about how best to man up to infertility.

CHAPTER ONE

Pete

The 20th October 2008 was the day I knew I was ready to become a father. My wife Emma and I had been working as doctors in Kuluva Hospital in north-west Uganda for the last three months and during our time there we had worked with and befriended many young children with Burkitt lymphoma, an aggressive, fast-growing type of cancer common in sub-Saharan African children that causes massive facial deformities. Kuluva Hospital was a regional centre for the disease and so many children and their families would stay for weeks at a time for their daily chemotherapy regimens. As part of our work we would do ward rounds and be involved in their treatments and then in the evening we would play with the kids, do activities and lead prayers and Bible stories. One group of children we became especially close to were Mparlo, Bupe, Kwami and a young boy called Eric. Before starting treatment, all the patients had a biopsy of the tumour, usually taken from their mouths under a general anaesthetic, and the sample would then be sent for histological analysis and diagnosis at Makerere University in Kampala. For one reason or another Eric missed having his biopsy and was started on his chemotherapy regime before a diagnosis was made (obviously not the best treatment by UK standards but common practice in rural Africa). Over the weeks, Mparlo, Bupe and Kwami's tumours all began to shrink but Eric's continued to grow around his neck and at the back of his throat. When it was noticed that Eric still hadn't had his biopsy he was booked in for surgery on the next available date. Although I'm not surgically trained, I was involved in assisting many operations during our time at Kuluva. Seeing that poor little boy in rag-like clothes sobbing in fear and pain after his operation and screaming for his 'Papa' was heart-breaking for me and I just scooped him up in my arms and carried him to where his father was waiting in the mid-afternoon heat. At that moment I felt for the first time a father's love for a child: to be a protector, rescuer, the feeling that you'd do anything to help them even if that meant dying for them, a sense of what God the ultimate Father must feel when he looks down on us. Although we knew Africa wasn't the right time or place to start trying for a family of our own, I knew I was ready to become a father when the time was right.

Emma and I met during my first year at university. We had so much in common and even our differences complemented each. We were both studying to be doctors and within months of meeting we both felt that the relationship was heading towards marriage. We got married in July 2005 when I was 22 and Emma 23 and it was a great celebration in front of friends and family at the church Emma had grown up in as a child and where we now go to as a family. We loved children and strangely had independently thought about having a family of both birth and adopted children, but we decided that we wanted to wait for a few years and spend time travelling, working overseas and getting through our medical exams. In 2009, having returned from working in Uganda, we decided the time was right to try to start our family.

How exciting it felt at the start! We'd finally got all our ducks in a row, ticked things off our 'to do list' and now we were ready for the baby . . . We knew the medical 'spiel' that most people get pregnant within a year and if not then most within two years so we tried to be relaxed as we started on this journey. But it quickly turned into a monthly rollercoaster of 'ovulation kits', body temperatures, 'fertile days', 'cervical mucus' and then the pregnancy tests which I soon dreaded, the sliding door moment where you hold your breath, hope for shrieks of joy and then realise the cycle continues for another month . . .

Didn't God know 'the plan'? One by one our friends around us all began to start having their own families, seemingly without any difficulties, and we became more and more convinced that we'd be in the group of one in seven UK couples who have difficulties conceiving.

Those negative niggles turned into negative words in our conversations, unaware and unacknowledging of the power in the words that we spoke.

'It's bound to be us who have problems.'

'It'd be just our luck that we won't be able to have children.'

The Bible says, 'The tongue has the power of life and death, and those who love it will eat its fruits' (Proverbs 18:21). And also, 'For as he thinks in his heart, so is he.' (Proverbs 23:7 NKJV).

Words are not just sounds produced by our vocal cords. Words have power. God created the world and universe with the power of his voice. Lies and unbelief were being spoken out of my mouth daily and the fruit of this quickly turned sour; I often found myself despondent, bitter, jealous and negative, unable to see beyond our circumstances.

Two years on and getting nowhere it felt like we were being left behind. It was like being at a train station with a ticket and suitcase packed and watching everyone else get on the train as they leave you to go on an amazing adventure. We decided it was time to go to our family doctor and get all the routine 'infertility tests' done. Box ticked and things all seemed fine; my 'boys' were healthy and all swimming in the right direction and Emma's hormone blood tests were all OK. 'Keep trying' was the advice.

This initially gave us a boost – everything's OK, nobody seems that worried, it will maybe just take longer for us. This boost was short lived, however, and I soon realised I needed to make a choice; a choice not to be defined by my circumstance or doctors' reports (positive or negative). I could not allow this to be all our life was about, making it into 'an idol' and allowing it to affect my marriage, friendships and ultimately my relationship with God.

It dawned on me that my 'great' faith actually wasn't all that great. It was the faith of a man whose life had been mostly plain sailing. I became a Christian aged seven but so far my faith had never really been put to the test and now cracks were starting to appear. In the pain and realness of our situation I had to 'man up' and do some soul searching into what I really believed about myself, our situation and God. There was no point singing the songs and praying the prayers if I didn't really believe what I was saying. I searched the Bible and prayed for answers, and over time God revealed his truth and his heart as a Father who loved me and cared for me, had good plans for me and would use all circumstances for his glory. I believe that this time of searching became the origins of this book.

I have to admit though, that at times going to church was difficult and careless comments from people stung us and seemed to rub salt into the wounds,

'You've been married eight years? When are you guys going to have a baby?'

'Don't you want kids?'

'Don't leave it too late. You're nearly thirty!'

At church, thoughts swirled through my mind,

'How can I sing that today?'

'How can they be preaching on that today? Doesn't God know what I'm going through?'

It's all too easy to give into the feelings of resentment and bitterness. But thankfully, over time as I understood more of God's goodness, I was able to allow him to comfort me and help bring me back (and he continually does) to that place of living a life of overcoming.

Eventually we were referred to see a fertility specialist at the hospital and after more tests and a diagnosis of endometriosis we were prescribed a drug called clomifene (Clomid) which stimulates the woman's ovaries to produce more eggs to increase the chance of a successful pregnancy. Surely this would do the trick, we thought. After another disappointing six months we still hadn't got pregnant and so we found ourselves back on the conveyor belt of more appointments, tests and opinions. Being a doctor didn't make this any easier; it felt frustratingly slow and inefficient, repeating tests we'd already had, and one doctor's opinion differing to another. In the midst of this confusion, coupled with increasing desperation, we could only cling on to the one constant in our life – God.

Eventually we were offered two different treatments: in vitro fertilisation (IVF), where eggs are removed from the woman and fertilised with a man's sperm to create an embryo which is then planted into the woman's uterus, or intrauterine insemination (IUI), where the woman is given hormone injections to stimulate the ovaries to produce more eggs, and at the time the eggs are released from the ovaries the man's sperm is injected through the woman's cervix into the uterus to try to fertilise the eggs. After researching and time in prayer we decided to have IUI treatment. This is a very personal choice for couples but we didn't feel comfortable with freezing embryos and discarding embryos that weren't growing well in IVF treatments. This can be a difficult decision for couples and needs prayer and careful discussions with your medical team. Whatever treatment (if any) you choose, one piece of advice we were given was to decide beforehand what treatments you felt comfortable with and to set a limit on the number of cycles. With IVF in particular there can be a huge financial cost (to say nothing of the emotional impact), with cycles in the UK costing around £5,000, and a real danger that, like the woman with a bleeding problem in Luke 8, you could spend all your money on doctors' bills.

Looking back, IUI was a very strange experience! I'll be blunt, producing a 'sample' on demand into a plastic pot in a dingy hospital room whilst avoiding looking at the 'adult' magazines 'helpfully' provided by the hospital and then handing it to a lab technician wasn't the greatest moment of my life! Holding my wife's hand with her legs in the air whilst a stranger injects your sperm into her cervix wasn't the way I envisioned starting a family either! After our fourth cycle we were getting disheartened and needed a breakthrough.

Through the ups and (mostly) downs of our journey we had become accustomed to starting again, regrouping and realigning our hearts and minds with God's truth and Scripture. We had to choose to put God before our circumstances despite the pain and feelings of hopelessness with our situation. As a husband I had to keep 'manning up' and allowing God to comfort me and give me the strength to keep persevering.

Emma had been reading a few books including a great book called *God's Plan for Pregnancy* by Nerida Walker; I'd really recommend reading it with your wife if you haven't read it. The book discussed about declaring Scriptures over your lives and in faith believing them as God's truth for your life and being encouraged by them. We felt this was something that might be helpful for us and during the next treatment cycle we chose and read over encouraging and healing Scriptures daily and we definitely felt an increase in peace, strength and closeness to God. Our faith was also boosted at a conference we went to where the speaker was talking about accelerated spiritual growth- something we'd both felt we were going through and then at the end of the conference someone we trusted and respected gave us a prophetic word that we were going to have our own birth children. The timing felt perfect for us to receive a miracle and we were so ready for it.

I'll never forget the morning when Emma finally had a positive pregnancy test. We were on a weekend break in the Peak District and Emma did her familiar secret, early morning pregnancy test whilst I pretended to be asleep, still daring to believe that our lives could change forever in the next few seconds. When the pregnancy test finally showed two pink lines it was incredible! Joy and relief rolled into one! When the time came for the ultrasound scan we were overwhelmed with happiness when we could see that tiny heart beating! Life felt amazing and all the years of pain seemed so distant. It felt such a relief, we could be a 'normal couple', our friends who had run out of encouraging things to say wouldn't need to feel awkward, people could cross us off their prayer lists and I wouldn't feel angry and bitter anymore.

When I started writing this book Emma was 10 weeks pregnant. I wanted to share what God had done for us and try to encourage other people in similar circumstances. We started telling our family and friends and it was just so encouraging to share our joy. Everyone was delighted – all their years of faithful prayers had been answered too!

One evening we'd just told the last of our close friends our good news. After dinner Emma noticed some light bleeding. The thought of us having a miscarriage had only briefly crossed our minds years before we'd even got pregnant but I confidently told Emma that after all we'd been through there was no way that this would happen to us.

Overnight things seemed fine and the next morning I went to work at 8 a.m as usual. At 9.15 a.m. I had a call from Emma to say that she'd had more bleeding so was coming to the hospital I was working at to get a scan. As we sat in the waiting room I felt excited that I was going to see our baby again and we started joking and talking about the future. We got called into the scanning room and I could see a baby-shaped blob on the screen and everything seemed fine. But the sonographer doing the scan turned to us and said the most devastating sentence anyone had ever told us: 'I'm really sorry but I can't find a heartbeat.'

Those words shook me to the core. I felt like I'd been hit by a train. We could not believe what we were hearing. Our miracle gift from God had died? Surely not. It didn't seem real. How could God have allowed this to happen? The lady stepped out of the room to give us some time and space alone.

'I don't believe this is going to happen' I said. 'Let's pray, I believe God can bring the baby back to life.'

When the sonographer came back I explained to her that we were Christians and that we'd been praying and believed God could change things. We asked if she could do the scan again because we believed the baby could have a heartbeat again. Reluctantly she agreed. If you were watching the story of our lives as a Hollywood blockbuster movie this is the part of the story where you might expect a miracle and our faith to be justified. Sadly not. As we peered at the grey and white images on the screen there was no miracle. We were stunned and devastated in equal measure.

The next few days my emotions swung wildly from crushing depression to wild hope that God could still bring our child back to life. We saw a video on YouTube about a couple from America whose baby died in the womb but then came back to life three weeks later and is now a perfectly healthy child. We know God doesn't have favourites so why couldn't that happen to us too and so we asked people to pray this for us. We named our baby Lazarus because the due date was Easter Sunday and if ever a baby was going to come back to life surely it would be our Easter baby!

We stayed strong; times alone, times together, reading, listening to music, praying with friends and going for walks in the park. Five days after we received our initial bad news Emma sadly passed our tiny baby – he was perfect. Weeping as we held him, we told him how much he was loved, that he was a miracle and how he had brought so much joy and encouragement to so many lives.

At the time this was the very worst thing that could have happened to me in my faith. Our Enemy knows us well and uses what he can against us when we are weak. Through the initial years of infertility, I sometimes wrongly felt that God didn't love me as much as everyone else and that our infertility was God's way of punishing me and that having to watch all our friends have a child, then second and third children was just another way of piling the misery on. After years of never quite daring to believe the Word of God as actual cast iron truth in the areas of our health and healing, we'd taken that step of faith into wholeheartedly believing God's truth. This was quickly challenged after we lost our baby and I experienced the darkest time of my life.

Initially God seemed tangibly close to us but as I kept questioning in my mind 'why us?', 'why our baby?', 'how can it say in the Bible there will be no miscarriage when it happened to us?' the doubts grew. That unshakeable trust that I had developed in God and his Word had been shattered and my whole world view and faith felt shaky.

'If these Bible verses aren't true, then maybe the rest of the Bible isn't true either?' I pondered. All these dark thoughts crept into my mind and there were times when I wanted nothing to do with God or his word. In my anger I even cancelled my direct debit to church (as if the creator of the universe would miss my tithe)!

On many occasions I accused God of standing by and watching our baby die and not caring, of watching in silence while our prayers were ignored and of making me look a fool when I said our baby could come back to life. One bad day I was sat alone at home angrily asking God again 'why us?' when he quietly whispered to me, 'Where do you think I was when my own innocent Son was crucified and died?'

That question stopped me dead and I began to well up. And then massive big sobs of realisation that God had to stand by powerlessly and watch his own son being crucified for my own sins. At a second's notice legions of angels could have been unleashed from heaven to stop it but God the Father chose not to. And the reason was because Jesus' death was the only way possible to redeem his sons and daughters, sons like me and you and daughters like Emma and your own wife. My sins meant that for me to be saved God had to watch his own innocent son be killed in the cruellest way imaginable. Sins of anger and lies that I was now pouring out to God. God was telling me he knew exactly how I was feeling because he had watched his own Son die. I was completely broken by this new understanding of God as a saving Father and that he had been standing with me through it all. Even now, years later, it still brings tears to my eyes. Such a powerful revelation of what an awesome Almighty Father we have!

Despite what I was learning about God, and the support of our friends and church I indulged in a lengthy pity party. In times of anger and despair I'd cry out statements such as, 'This is ruining my life!'

The truth was my life was being ruined but only because I was allowing my response to the miscarriage to ruin my relationship with God. I was feeling angry and frustrated at my church small group, I purposely avoided friends who had families and allowed friendships that had been built over years to drift away. But who was that hurting? Only myself, and it did really hurt.

In the weeks and months after our miscarriage I tried to reduce my frustrations by doing as much sport as I could. I took up triathlons and started training as hard as I could. In truth it was a much healthier way of dealing with my anger compared to drink, drugs or whatever other vices you could be tempted with, but compared to turning to God it was ultimately futile. A few days before I took part in a duathlon in the Peak District I heard our pastor preach at our men's Bible study and one of the verses he used was Romans 11:29: 'God's gifts and his call are irrevocable.'

I couldn't believe my pastor had said that,

'How insensitive,' I inwardly seethed. 'You were only at our home a few weeks ago when we were so distraught and now you're telling me God's gifts are irrevocable. How can that be true when our baby died?'

That verse really started to bug me. As I was pedalling over a steep climb on the bike leg of the duathlon those words were driving me mad with frustration. In the midst of my annoyance I felt the calm voice of God in my mind:

'Your baby is with me in eternity. You'll see him again one day. My gifts *are* irrevocable.'

It's amazing how God can speak to people. On a beautiful crisp October morning God had proved to me how his Word remains true despite the facts of our situation. God's gifts are irrevocable. I'll see our baby again one day, and also for eternity.

Twice God had spoken to me in a powerful way and I knew that my choice was to continue living my life in the pity party or to man up and get back to being the man God created me to be and the husband that Emma needed me to be (and restarting my direct debit monthly tithe!). I chose the latter and although it's been far from easy, as evidenced by the years taken to finish this book, I'm so glad I made the choice to come wholeheartedly back to God.

A large part of turning back to God was learning to trust his Word again even though it was hard and our circumstances often didn't line up with what we were reading. At one point I thought maybe God just didn't want us to have children but through studying God's Word we can see that isn't his intention and a big part of God's plan for us all is to be part of families and have children. Even God's first recorded words that he speaks to humans were 'Be fruitful and increase in number; fill the earth and subdue it' (Genesis 1:28).

It was through the first sin and the fall of Adam (Genesis 3) that sickness and death came into the world, and infertility is just another part of that. The knowledge that God does want us to be fruitful and have children has been a great encouragement to me.

My journey's focus shifted from the goal of simply having a child and being a father, to the fulfilment of living a life that is fully surrendered to God and living in the freedom God brings in every area of my life come what may. I was determined not to miss out on any more of God's goodness and blessing in life by holding onto the pain and loss I had experienced. Over the years we started to pray and think more and more about adoption and the opportunity to give children a loving home.

If your heart is set on having 'your own' birth children then adoption may feel like a 'second-best' choice, but it simply isn't. As we'll see, God used the adoption of children into new families for some of the most important men and women in the Old and New Testaments. Ultimately, God's plan for mankind's salvation depends on a man who was adopted and that in turn allows us to be adopted into God's eternal family.

So, to pick up our personal journey from where we left off, we'd switched our mindset from being solely focussed on having a baby to making peace with God, choosing to keep trusting him – even though things didn't make sense to us – and trying to live overcoming lives. As I've already said, we'd always wanted to have adopted children in our family. After years of infertility a familiar verse spoke to us again in a fresh way: 'The thief comes only to steal and kill and destroy; I have come that they may have life, and have it to the full' (John 10:10).

You may think that choosing to adopt was giving up on God and hypocritical after everything I've said and written about in this book so far. I wholeheartedly believe all the stories of overcoming infertility in the Bible and I know God can and still does work miracles today. However, we will never fully understand God, nor do we know why people suffer, why young people and children die from cancer or why some couples never have birth children. God in his grace gave us the opportunity to adopt and I'm so glad we did. I'll never let my own personal circumstances dictate what I know to be true about my Heavenly Father and his nature. Bill Johnson, the lead pastor of Bethel Church in Redding, California, puts it like this: 'I will not sacrifice my knowledge of the goodness of God on the altar of human reasoning so I can have an explanation for a seemingly unanswered prayer.'

My wise grandmother's favourite Scripture was this:

Trust in the LORD with all your heart
  and lean not on your own understanding;
in all your ways submit to him,
  and he will make your paths straight.

(Proverbs 3:5–6)

The key is to trust and not rely on our own fallible understanding. We believed the Enemy had robbed us of being a family for too long and we also knew that there were lots of children who needed loving parents. I can't go into any details of our childrens' adoptions but we knew when we read their profiles they were meant to be in our family. Trust me when I say it wasn't an easy process, but as always God helped us through the testing times of the journey. We are now the proud parents of three beautiful children!

As with all journeys of faith there is always more to learn and areas to grow in, more questions to ask and more answers to receive. I wanted to share with you some of those key lessons that I have learnt along the way (sometimes the hard way!) in the hope they may help you too.

Waiting well

The years spent waiting are really difficult. Thankfully we have in Joseph – the man with the 'Technicolour Dream Coat' – an example from the Bible of a man who waited well.

The chief cupbearer, however, did not remember Joseph; he forgot him . . . When two full years had passed, Pharaoh had a dream. (Genesis 40: 23 and Genesis 41:1)

What must Joseph have thought during those two years in the Egyptian prison? Falsely accused and wrongly imprisoned, he'd trusted God all those years, correctly interpreted the dreams of Pharaoh's baker and cupbearer, and yet was still rotting in the jail like a common criminal. Who could blame him for wanting to give up? I know I would have felt like giving up! If you'd taken a snapshot of Joseph's life at that moment you'd have no option but to conclude that his life was an utter failure: rejected by his family, sold into slavery, left in prison and now it seemed God had totally forgotten and abandoned him.

That's how I often felt – forgotten and abandoned. Maybe that's how you're feeling now. You've been trying to start (or add to) your family for years, you trust in God's Word and still nothing changes. Maybe you're struggling with your faith, you've got an anger problem, you could be struggling with addictions to drugs, gambling, alcohol or pornography. A snapshot picture of your life would be one of failure too. But when we read the story of Joseph we can gloss over those two years in jail because we know that's not how his story ends. God does remember him and he goes on to become second in charge to Pharaoh, saving his whole family in the process.

When you're going through the hard times of life you've got to remember that this is not the whole story, this isn't how the journey ends. God wants to bless you and he has an awesome plan for your life, and in two, three, four years (who knows how many years' time) you'll be looking back and saying that was a hard time but God was with me through it.

Thoughts

As I've already said, our thoughts are incredibly powerful. When negative thoughts of doubt, despair, anger or jealousy get into your mind you can quickly spiral into depression and just like that your walk with God goes astray. The key to combatting this is first to recognise that the thoughts you are believing are just lies or that you are looking at things from a worldly perspective rather than God's, then secondly to allow God to replace these thoughts with his truth. Paul teaches on this in his second letter to the Corinthians:

The weapons we fight with are not the weapons of the world. On the contrary, they have divine power to demolish strongholds. We demolish arguments and every pretension that sets itself up against the knowledge of God, and we take captive every thought to make it obedient to Christ. (2 Corinthians 10:4–5)

God is gracious and meets us where we're at but he doesn't want us to allow the pity party to become an 'all-nighter'. Whenever a negative thought comes into our minds we need to learn to recognise the lie before we start believing it. It's natural to have negative feelings and thoughts when you are going through infertility (and I wouldn't believe you if you said you didn't!) but we don't want them to become our default setting.

For example, I often fell into the thought pattern of thinking God didn't love me as much as others or I didn't deserve to be blessed as much as my friends. When I began to recognise this happening I saw them for the lies they were and was able to replace these thoughts with the truth. I would read through parts of the Bible that show God is a good Father who wants to give us good things and has no favourites, which over time helped me renew my heart and mind.

Going through the fire

Throughout the Bible God ultimately saved his people from hard times and their enemies but they still had to go through those character defining moments alongside Him. Jesus didn't say that following him would be easy and trouble free. On the contrary he said, 'In this world you will have trouble. But take heart! I have overcome the world' (John 16:33).

So from this we know that in the Christian life we *will* have troubles but we also know that God has promised, 'I will never leave you nor forsake you' (Joshua 1:5)

I've prayed many times that God would take our infertility away from us but so far this hasn't happened. Sometimes it feels like God isn't there or he doesn't care but the truth is that he always is.

My absolute favourite story in the Bible is the story of three friends; Shadrach, Meshach and Abednego. The story in Daniel chapters 1-3 tells of the friends being taken from their homeland into captivity in Babylon after Jerusalem had been devastated and they were forced to serve the evil King Nebuchadnezzar. What a picture of desperation and defeat and yet these men along with Daniel refuse to give up on God and in that dark place they bring glory to him. In chapter 3 all the citizens are ordered by King Nebuchadnezzar to bow down and worship a golden statue, but the three friends refuse. They knew refusing could cost their lives but they had faith that God could save them from death, but even if he didn't they still wouldn't bow down and worship the statue!

> If we are thrown into the blazing furnace, the God we serve is able to deliver us from it, and he will deliver us from Your Majesty's hand. But even if he does not, we want you to know, Your Majesty, that we will not serve your gods or worship the image of gold you have set up.
>
> *(Daniel 3:17–18)*

That's the kind of man I want to be – standing up for what's right no matter the cost. Shadrach, Meshach and Abednego are the kind of friends I'd love to have (and do have) and the kind of friend I aspire to be like. Even though God didn't prevent them from being thrown into the furnace he was still there with them in the flames: 'Look! I see four men walking around in the fire, unbound and unharmed, and the fourth looks like a son of the gods' (Daniel 3:25).

There's lots we can learn from this story of three men 'going through the fire'. Firstly, the very fact that they weren't prevented from being thrown into the furnace shows that God doesn't always stop bad things happening to us – but if they do he can always bring good from it: 'And we know that in all things God works for the good of those who love him, who have been called according to his purpose' (Romans 8:28).

Secondly, when the three men were in the furnace their hands were untied and free. We can often feel like our hands are tied and we're helpless in the face of infertility but God can free us from its grip on us. God doesn't want us to be living with our hands tied like slaves to the frustration and disappointment that it brings. Like the three friends, God is standing with us in the fire and has set us free so we don't have to be governed by our circumstances. Paul tells us, 'It is for freedom that Christ has set us free. Stand firm, then, and do not let yourselves be burdened again by a yoke of slavery' (Galatians 5:1).

I feel like my own infertility battle has at times kept me a slave to it. Jesus came to set us free from this and while he may not give you what you want immediately, he wants us to be set free to live as overcomers who reflect his love and ultimately lead others to him.

I love how these verses in Romans show us how God works in our struggles:

Not only so, but we also glory in our sufferings, because we know that suffering produces perseverance; perseverance, character; and character, hope. And hope does not put us to shame, because God's love has been poured out into our hearts through the Holy Spirit, who has been given to us.

(Romans 5:3-5)

It's certainly true that the hard 'in the fire' times are when we grow the most and I know if I hadn't had to go on this journey then I would still most likely be that man with a surface-deep faith and living my 'normal' life.

Steven Furtick, pastor of Elevation Church in Charlotte, North Carolina, puts it like this:

Sometimes your greatest testimony is that you went through fire but don't even smell like smoke.

Now there's a challenge!

Doing things in your own strength

Sometimes it felt like if I prayed more, fasted more or studied the Bible more that it would somehow 'persuade' God to give me children. We often feel we need to 'do' something when we feel helpless and hopeless, and these things can all be part of a healthy Christian life, but there's nothing we can 'do' in our own strength to increase God's provision for us.

Everything Jesus' did for us on the cross means the battle against sickness (including infertility) and death has already been won. In Paul's letter to the church in Ephesus on the armour of God he tells us we simply need to stand our ground. We don't need to 'win' the battle ourselves, all we need to do is 'stand'.

Finally, be strong in the Lord and in his mighty power. Put on the full armour of God, so that you can take your *stand* against the devil's schemes. For our struggle is not against flesh and blood, but against the rulers, against the authorities, against the powers of this dark world and against the spiritual forces of evil in the heavenly realms. Therefore put on the full armour of God, so that when the day of evil comes, you may be able to *stand* your ground, and after you have done everything, to *stand. Stand* firm then, with the belt of truth buckled around your waist, with the breastplate of righteousness in place, and with your feet fitted with the readiness that comes from the gospel of peace. In addition to all this, take up the shield of faith, with which you can extinguish all the flaming arrows of the evil one. Take the helmet of salvation and the sword of the Spirit, which is the word of God. And pray in the Spirit on all occasions with all kinds of prayers and requests. With this in mind, be alert and always keep on praying for all the Lord's people.

(Ephesians 6:10–18, emphasis mine)

It's only after putting on our armour that we can stand, and this is where reading the Bible, prayer, fasting and growing in our faith are important. There have definitely been times when I have felt 'I can't stand (this) anymore, God!' This is when I have been so thankful to have faithful friends surrounding me, who have 'stood' with me in prayer and helped me keep 'standing'.

I know it can feel humiliating as a guy to be vulnerable with others but make sure you man up and get yourself surrounded by some more of his warriors to stand alongside you in this battle.

Your best mate's having a(nother) baby

When you face this situation you've got a choice: act like a jerk or act like a best friend! Unfortunately, there have been times when I'm ashamed to say I've acted like a jerk. If he's your best mate chances are he's a good guy so he'll understand that you may find it difficult, but the times when I've rejoiced with my friends have been the most rewarding and so beneficial to the friendship.

As you go through your journey you may meet other couples going through the same struggles. That can be a great source of encouragement but also difficulties can arise when a couple gets their breakthrough and the others are left still waiting. These Bible verses can help in these situations:

> Praise be to the God and Father of our Lord Jesus Christ, the Father of compassion and the God of all comfort, who comforts us in all our troubles, so that we can comfort those in any trouble with the comfort we ourselves receive from God.
>
> *(2 Corinthians 1:3–4)*

And also:

> Rejoice with those who rejoice; mourn with those who mourn.
>
> *(Romans 12:15)*

Hospital appointments

You need to be well prepared for going to hospital appointments as these can be a source of stress and tension between you and your wife. The chances are that the medical staff will speak the medical facts to you, which may not always be in line with God's truth for your life.

On one occasion we'd got the time wrong for an appointment and were really late, which then lead to a big argument in the car. When we eventually arrived at the hospital, we couldn't find a spot to park – you can imagine the stress! At our appointment we received unexpected bad test results which hit us hard as we weren't in the best place to face such news. You're much more likely to be victorious when you approach these things from a position of strength based on God's Word and provision. We were trying to overcome these setbacks from a position of weakness where we'd been arguing and not standing strong together and so it took weeks to recover from this. You've got to be wise and prepare yourselves when going to medical appointments so you can stand together in God's hope and peace. Maybe try listening to worship music or praying together beforehand, whatever it takes for you to enter your appointment in a position of strength.

It is not only disappointing medical results and opinions, you can also be faced with negative attitudes of staff who may see things differently to you. I remember being taken aback by one nurse who kept asking what we would do when this treatment didn't work! She herself was pregnant and she appeared bigger and bigger over the months of our treatment! She couldn't quite get her head round the fact we were still standing in hope that the treatment *was* going to be successful this time. All I could do in that situation was to take a deep breath and pray for her to have a healthy pregnancy and a safe delivery . . . despite the temptation for an angry outburst!

Miscarriage

This is a devastating setback to experience during infertility; a pregnancy so longed for and that chance of finally being a parent (again) being robbed so cruelly from you. This is exactly how we felt.

We know God is a good Father who gives blessings, does not cause sickness and that miscarriage was never part of his plan for His people: 'None will miscarry or be barren' (Exodus 23:26). Sadly in this world sickness and miscarriage are a common occurrence. It is estimated to happen in about one in every eight pregnancies and most miscarriages are not caused by anything the mother did neither could they be prevented. Many Christians, myself included, believe life begins at conception and so any unborn child is still precious and loved by God, and this has brought us so much comfort.

> Before I formed you in the womb I knew you, before you were born I set you apart.
>
> *(Jeremiah 1:5)*

We know that God is the ultimate creator of life, as he has been since the beginning of time, and that he alone knows the number of our days on earth. He creates every child and watches them grow, delighting in them and valuing every single day of their life, however short.

> For you created my inmost being;
>   you knit me together in my mother's womb.
> I praise you because I am fearfully and wonderfully made;
>   your works are wonderful,
> I know that full well.
> My frame was not hidden from you
>   when I was made in the secret place,
>   when I was woven together in the depths of the earth.
> Your eyes saw my unformed body;
>   all the days ordained for me were written in your book
>   before one of them came to be.
>
> *(Psalm 139:13–16)*

Even though we lost our first child I know one day I'll see him again in heaven. One of King David's sons died as a small infant and in his grief he expressed his belief that he would see him again one day: 'I will go to him, but he will not return to me' (2 Samuel 12:23).

If you and your wife lose a baby it is completely understandable to be angry at an all-powerful God who could have prevented it, but as I learned it is far better to turn to a God who also knows the pain of losing his only Son and who promises to give us peace and comfort in our distress (2 Corinthians 1:3–4).

One of my hopes for this book was that through some of my experiences I may be of help and a comfort for those struggling in the same way. I know in turn that God will also use your journey to be a comfort for others too.

Facebook

Don't get me wrong, I've nothing against Facebook or any other social media but I do think it can make the struggle with infertility more painful. It's a great way to keep in touch with friends and family but it can also be a distraction in our walk with God. A recent study showed that people in the UK spent (wasted?!) on average 1 hour and 20 minutes on social media a day. How long do we spend reading our Bibles? Now that's a sobering thought!

We decided to come off Facebook for a while because seeing posts of ultrasound scans, constant announcements, baby talk and pictures was not hugely helpful when we were often feeling vulnerable. The timing was usually impeccable: a negative pregnancy test for us followed by a flurry of Facebook new baby announcements. It wasn't something that was 'building me up' any longer and often in the early days just added fuel to my pity party.

Facebook (or Fakebook as I've heard it described) is often being used as the 'highlights' reel of people's lives. Only showing the pictures that make you out to be living the perfect life creates a false impression that can leave others feeling depressed. You'll never see the 20 bad pictures before the 'perfect one' and no one ever posts a selfie of them arguing with their spouse or their children fighting each other or having a tantrum!

We can all develop an unhealthy obsession with social media and so if it's making you or your wife feel depressed I'd highly recommend cancelling your account or limiting the time you spend on it. Personally, we've found that to be one of the best things we've done in this journey.

Comparing our lives to other people's is never a healthy thing to do and usually makes us either depressed and jealous or prideful and judgemental. Basically, don't compare yourself to others – you've got your own job to do and that's to follow God's path for your own life.

Prayer and praise

On this journey of overcoming infertility you may have started by praying with your wife, but as time goes on perhaps you have begun to share your struggles with close friends and family or your small group, asking them all to pray too. As things feel more desperate and the battle is seemingly bigger than you first thought you may end up going through your church hierarchy to the assistant pastor and then senior pastor for their prayer and support. Then there's the Christian conference, healing retreat or asking a famous or 'celebrity' Christian to pray for you, all with the hope that their prayers might 'work'.

I'm not criticising this way of thinking, and in fact we did most of these things too, including getting prayer when visiting a friend at Bethel Church in California (a church famous for seeing numerous miracles). There's nothing wrong with asking people to pray for us; indeed we should be doing that and also praying for others too. The danger is that we can start to look to people who we think are 'special' or 'super spiritual' for our miracle rather than God.

It reminds me of the father who took his epileptic son to the disciples. I'm pretty sure he would have asked God to heal his son and probably would have asked his friends, family and leaders in the synagogue to pray too. In desperation he takes his son to the disciples but even they are unable to heal him. Finally, he brings him to Jesus:

Jesus asked the boy's father, 'How long has he been like this?'

'From childhood,' he answered. 'It has often thrown him into fire or water to kill him. But if you can do anything, take pity on us and help us.'

'"If you can'?" said Jesus. 'Everything is possible for one who believes.'

Immediately the boy's father exclaimed, 'I do believe; help me overcome my unbelief!'

When Jesus saw that a crowd was running to the scene, he rebuked the impure spirit. 'You deaf and mute spirit,' he said, 'I command you, come out of him and never enter him again.'

The spirit shrieked, convulsed him violently and came out. The boy looked so much like a corpse that many said,

'He's dead.' But Jesus took him by the hand and lifted him to his feet, and he stood up.

(Mark 9:21–27)

Ultimately, it's God alone who has the power to heal and we need to find our own way to keep looking upwards to him. The words of the father in this story sum up perfectly for me the tension we all face in looking to God for healing: 'I do believe; help me overcome my unbelief!'

It's that paradox that we believe and yet doubt at the same time. It's that desperate cry to God to help us have more faith to keep on believing change is possible even when we don't see healing immediately.

Prayer isn't only a list of requests. God wants to know how we are feeling, our hurts and fears as well as our thanks and praise. In Psalms there are many examples of songs (prayers) where the writer starts by pouring out his heart to God and then by the end declaring truth, victory and praise to God.

Certain worship songs became Emma's and my own anthems for the different seasons we journeyed through and the time I spent in praise listening to them and talking to God really did refresh my soul and give me peace and comfort. I really encourage you to find your own anthems and use them to talk to God.

We must also never forget that prayer is a two-way conversation and listening is key. There is so much God will be doing in your life beyond your longing for infertility breakthrough and you can't lose sight of that.

So that's the end of our journey into parenthood. I hope you've been helped in some way by our story, there were some painful and disappointing times but lots of spiritual growth, our marriage certainly felt stronger after all we'd been through together and then finally the incredible blessings of our three children!

CHAPTER TWO

Ben

names anonymised

My name is Ben and I am 30 years old. I became a Christian nine years ago, during my final year at university. I work for a social welfare charity in Swansea, happily married to Lydia and we have a three-year-old little boy called Joseph and a two-week-old baby girl!

Before Lydia and I were married she explained to me that she had always had an irregular menstrual cycle caused by polycystic ovary syndrome (PCOS) and that might make having children difficult. I confessed to her that for some strange reason I had always had a sense, whenever I thought about children, that I might not be guaranteed children naturally, and for some reason I even doubted my own fertility at that point. For me, it was not a problem; I loved Lydia and would support her whatever lay ahead. We often talked about our willingness to look into adoption, because we recognised the great need out there for mums and dads. We even attended an information event about adoption early into married life but both felt it was too soon.

Two years passed and Lydia started treatment for PCOS and so began having more regular menstrual cycles. The drug she had to take seemingly got everything working as it should and we hoped this would help us start a family. However, God had other plans. One morning, out of the blue, Lydia woke me up after a particularly vivid dream she had experienced. In this dream she strongly felt like God was asking her to look after his children. He kindly and gently asked her if we would adopt and be the parents of a little boy. After Lydia relayed the full dream back to me, I just knew that we should start looking into it. This was the start of one of the most amazing journeys, and we really felt like we were walking in step with God's will for our lives.

Adoption is a challenging journey but we had some great friends who had been through it themselves and mentored us through the process. It was nothing short of miraculous. From the day we registered our interest, to the day we took Joseph home, was exactly nine months. God blew us away in so many ways during the process, confirming time and time again that he was in control. Joseph was seven months old when we took him home. Even more miraculously, three years later Lydia gave birth to our daughter Lily.

The day we found out Lydia was pregnant came just after a conversation we had had about having more children. Despite attempts to adopt for a second time, it seemed to be more challenging and the door kept closing on us. We discussed looking at restarting the medical process and treatment again but agreed that we would not do that and trust God's timing instead. His timing was amazing as later that same day we were absolutely delighted to discover that she was in fact already pregnant!

God saw our hearts for adoption, and even though we had forgotten about it, he prompted us through a dream. It was not until Joseph had been home with us that we realised that his name (not given by us) was the name of two men in the Bible who heard God speak through dreams!

A really important Scripture for us was this:

For you, God, tested us; you refined us like silver. You brought us into prison and laid burdens on our backs. You let people ride over our heads; we went through fire and water, but you brought us to a place of abundance.

(Psalm 66:10–12)

God gave us these verses at a conference, a few years ago. It was at a time when Lydia was working in prison as part of the chaplaincy team and had an accident at home. She had fallen down the stairs and suffered three prolapsed disks in her spine. She was completely incapacitated for a while and in lots of pain for a long time. It was a challenging time, but through this Scripture we knew God saw all that, and we knew that something good was going to come from it because he promised abundance, which we held on to as a promise. He was refining us like the silversmith refines silver, waiting to see his reflection in the precious metal before he knows it is ready. We were being refined through fire in his image, even through the midst of a difficult and painful time. When we went through the adoption process a while later, this challenging season was looked on really favourably when we were scrutinised and assessed. Despite our young age, it showed resilience and our ability to overcome a really difficult time in our married lives together. Who would have thought it?

I believe God loves adoption and is part of his plan for mankind. He invites us all to be adopted into his family as full heirs and co-heirs with his son Jesus. We receive all this when we invite Jesus to be in our lives and accept his saving grace through his death and resurrection. It seems to me that our journey with Joseph is almost a microcosm of this divine truth, because he is fully our son and always will be. Not just in legal terms, but so much more. I have learnt and been reminded that God uses adoption for our redemption, and I think we should not be surprised when he calls us to do the same, whatever the circumstances, because it really is in step with the Father's heart.

I sometimes have doubts and wonder about my effectiveness as a disciple of Christ. However, I know that God has given us a child who I have the privilege and responsibility to disciple. If that is my main calling in life, then it is a precious and worthwhile one. I might not be responsible for the evangelisation of thousands but that makes my call no less important. I have no doubt God has put a call on Joseph's life; this is so apparent in how he came to be with us, and who knows how God will use his life in the fullness of time. Greater things I am sure! That is not just a proud father speaking!

So many people we meet say they would like to adopt but, sadly, very few act on it. I would encourage you to think and pray about it. Do not overthink it though, because you will discover many obstacles and reasons why you shouldn't adopt. I believe that choosing to adopt is a way we can put our faith into action. If you believe God is calling you to it, then hold on to that even when everything and everyone else may seem against it. Trust in him.

CHAPTER THREE

Chris

names anonymised

I'm Chris, I'm 33 and I live in Liverpool with my wife Kate. I first asked Jesus into my life when I was five years old. My grandparents and uncle had just been killed in a road accident and I was asking questions about where they had gone and what happens after you die. I knew I wanted to be with Jesus after I died so, with my mum, I prayed and asked Jesus into my life.

I quietly rebelled a bit through high school and was often a 'part time' Christian. Although I never lost my faith, I knew I needed to start afresh and give every area of my life and my future to God, which I did when I moved up to Edinburgh to study aged 18.

I met Kate at church four years later; we were both helping on an Alpha course and soon after we went with a mission team to Zambia. We got to know each other whilst helping villagers build a healthcare clinic in the day and at night around the campfire under the stars. After a couple of years, we got engaged on a rainy day in North Wales and then married the following summer in Hull. After various jobs, including teaching and working for a charity in Uganda for a year, we felt God call us to lead an Eden team with the Message Trust in Liverpool. We knew God was calling us to settle in Liverpool and we decided now would be the perfect time to start a family. I was cautious and a bit nervous about whether I'd make a good dad. Though I have a great relationship with my dad now, it wasn't always so good growing up. It felt like a lot of change in a short time, but Kate didn't want to wait any longer and after praying it felt like it was the right time.

After the first month we excitedly took a pregnancy test, nervous and expectant that it would be positive. When it wasn't, there was a tiny bit of disappointment but also some relief that we had more time to get used to the idea.

Another month came and went and we reassured ourselves after some Googling that this was totally normal. After a few more months we gradually became more and more disappointed and frustrated. We were reading lots of different advice but knew that we couldn't get any medical help until we had been trying for a while. After a year we went to the doctors together and began fertility tests.

During this time there were a few moments when I felt God speak to me about having children. Someone praying for me said they had the word 'fruitful' for me, which I took to mean having children, and another said they saw a picture of a stork delivering a baby to our house in Liverpool – random, but again I thought, 'I'll have that one too'! Neither individual had known what we were going through. We both went for prayer at a Christian festival called New Wine and a wise elderly man faithfully prayed that we would have a baby by the same time next year.

I've found it hard in the past to hear God on things that I longed for; it's easy to convince yourself either way that God has spoken, doubt that he has or twist what he's saying to fit what you really want. The long months of waiting overshadowed those moments where we felt God might be speaking and giving us hope, but still the hope hung on.

We had now been waiting 18 months and by this time it was getting really hard and affecting both of us in different ways. Kate was feeling it by far the most and I wasn't always as sympathetic as I could or should have been. It became harder especially for Kate to be happy for friends around us who one by one were having children. We'd spent time with communities, families and individuals who had been through horrific suffering, both in Africa and on our own estate. We knew that not having children wasn't nearly the hardest thing to cope with, but the longer we waited the bigger the issue became and the more our lives, conversations and prayers focused on it.

We had great support from friends at church who were going through similar challenges and so could share what we felt and pray together. We told our parents, which was quite hard to do, but they too were very supportive and understanding.

It was at about this time when we got the news that my youngest brother's fiancée, who our family had known since she was born, had cancer. They were due to get married in the summer but her illness rapidly worsened. We were able to spend some time with both of them before she became very ill. One of the last times we spoke to her, she said that while we had been praying for her a lot she really wanted to be praying for us. So we told her we really wanted to have children.

It was while we were getting ready to travel to Yorkshire the morning before their wedding that Kate decided to quickly take a pregnancy test, so that it wasn't at the back of her mind with everything else going on. We were just about to leave when she told me she was pregnant! Not really knowing what to do with the information we quickly prayed and set off, only to find out three hours later that very sadly my brother's fiancée had passed away that morning. It was an incredibly difficult and sad time, but also strangely beautiful and special, turning what had been planned as a wedding into a thanksgiving service for her life. It was a huge privilege to be with the wider family for her funeral a while later and spend a day being together and remembering her.

We suppressed any excitement about being pregnant until our first scan and were able to tell our parents, family and friends, which brought new hope and joy into some dark months. As we got closer to the birth, we got more and more excited and a bit scared about our lives changing and being responsible for a whole new life when we couldn't even keep house plants alive! We knew what we would call the baby if it was a girl but couldn't think of any boy's names we liked or could agree on. One night, Kate woke me up saying she'd just had a dream where God told her what to call the baby if it was a boy! I asked what it was but Kate couldn't remember and she didn't remember for weeks! The name was Cayden, one that we would not have considered or chosen ourselves. This name was confirmed a few weeks before the birth when we were at a prayer day for the Message Trust. The drummer in the worship band came over at lunchtime and said while he was drumming God gave him a word for us that our baby would stand on our shoulders in terms of his faith, and that the baby would be an amazing man of prayer and a mighty warrior for God. We knew Cayden meant 'mighty warrior' but we also knew that women could be great warriors too so didn't want to assume anything!

Cayden's birth was incredible and very special for both of us. We are very grateful to God for answering our prayers and are careful not to take Cayden for granted, whilst at the same time avoiding being too precious or protective of him. He is an incredibly happy boy who has brought a lot of joy to everyone who spends time with him, which quite often includes complete strangers out shopping or on the street.

When Cayden was one and Kate had stopped breastfeeding him we decided we should start trying again as it had taken so long to get pregnant. We prayed for more children and talked it through. We thought it would be much easier if we had to wait again as Cayden was a big distraction, as well as a sign of hope. We also hoped things would be simpler the second time and many people told us it would probably be much quicker and easier. It wasn't. The months started to pass and we began to feel like we were back in the same frustrating place. Despite Cayden being very happy and knowing no different, we'd watch him playing by himself. Kate and I both have siblings who we are close to, and we longed for Cayden to have a brother or sister to play with. Friends and family were continuing to have more children. Praying and supporting other friends who were still waiting for a baby became trickier as we now had Cayden.

After trying for six or seven months Kate had a positive pregnancy test, though it was faint. Things progressed well for a few weeks but on Kate's birthday we found out it was an ectopic pregnancy (when the baby develops in the fallopian tubes and not the womb). This was a big blow and really upsetting, especially for Kate. We received a lot of love and support from church, friends and family and grieved the loss. This was different to the numb, constant background grief of waiting to get pregnant and the regular disappointment and frustration that we began to expect each month, this felt much harder and heavier.

Doctors told us that while the medication Kate was on for the ectopic pregnancy worked through her body we were not to try to conceive again for at least three months. This was another hard thing to take but did give us a strange sense of relief and rest over the first month. But time began to run away and Cayden was growing up fast and beginning to ask for a brother or sister like many of his friends had.

We looked more and more seriously at adoption and fostering and saw both good and bad examples of families where adoption had really worked and other cases where it was difficult. We had also supported a struggling mum when we first moved to our estate who had had all her children taken from her which was heart breaking to see and gave us another and very different perspective on the process. We really wanted a bigger family, naturally if possible, but if not then we trusted God would make it happen one way or another.

Earlier in the year, a friend had given me a prophetic word that our children would stand on our shoulders in terms of their faith and being missionaries to the urban poor. When he said children he stopped and reiterated, saying not our spiritual children (as in those we had helped find Jesus for themselves) but our blood children. I got very excited about him saying blood children as I was sure this meant we were going to have more than one! However, my friend also stresses, when teaching on prophecy, that you should avoid prophecy about babies or marriage as it can often be very unhelpful and at the time he hadn't realised how I had taken what he'd said!

After trying for over a year, and not having had any follow-up after the ectopic pregnancy, we went back to the doctors and started a fresh round of fertility tests. Kate had a number of scans and was sent from one doctor to the next before finally seeing a consultant a week before Christmas. The consultant explained that Kate would need to have an operation to remove her fallopian tube as it had been very badly damaged from the ectopic pregnancy. There were some other smaller complications and the consultant said that we would need to look into IVF. When Kate explained that we already had one child, she was surprised and bluntly said that this was more than likely the end of the road in terms of naturally having children. Kate had seen the consultant alone whilst I looked after Cayden and within the space of her ten-minute appointment went from being hopeful to leaving totally dejected. We had the evening in together and Kate said the consultant had happened to mention as she was being scanned that an egg was about to be released. This seemed to add salt to the wound at the time but we decided to pray, and we determined that we would only accept God's word and not that of the consultant. Well, later that month Kate took another pregnancy test as she was feeling ill and sure enough she was pregnant!

Even more than before we didn't want to get excited; it was amazing but we also knew things were not right in Kate's body and this could be quite dangerous. We kept quiet and subdued and continued to pray, gradually asking people who we knew understood and could trust to pray for us too. Eventually we had an early positive scan and were able to tell more friends and family. Due to having been through all the highs and lows of trying to start a family and knowing so many people who were still struggling to start a family, we didn't make a big fuss publicly, but privately we were overjoyed at another miracle life beginning.

My older brother and sister-in-law had recently had their second baby and then my other brother and sister-in-law announced they were expecting their first. Everything was looking great at that time! We were looking forward to a big family celebration of my dad's retirement, my parents' 40th wedding anniversary and the influx of grandchildren.

However, totally unexpectedly, at the start of the summer my mum, who was healthy and active and had never been to hospital except to give birth to me and my brothers, had a stroke and was rushed to hospital. After some time in hospital and then at home, she had made good progress and was back walking and gearing up for a family holiday.

Two days after she was discharged I got a call saying she had been rushed back into hospital. It wasn't another stroke but she was very unwell. After further tests the doctors told us that she had secondary cancer of the liver and spleen. She continued to deteriorate and sadly died a few weeks after our second baby was born.

One thing we have learnt while waiting for children is that God's timing is perfect. It doesn't feel like that when you're going through it and it hasn't in the past, but we know and trust it is. We're all heartbroken that we're not going to be together and that Mum isn't here to see and help the kids grow up. She was an incredible, inspiring, creative and very loving Grannie and leaves a huge and painful gap because she brought so much joy and love. We have a lot to be thankful for and know we've experienced so much love and joy because of Jesus in our lives. He will help us through the storms and the hard times ahead as well as the joy of new life and everything it brings.

I don't remember much in terms of key Bible passages or advice people have given me over the last few years. What I do know is that I wouldn't want to have gone through any of the bad or the good times without God, and the closer we can be to Jesus each day through the Bible, worship, community and prayer the better we'll celebrate the highs and weather the storms.

Let us hold unswervingly to the hope we profess, for he who promised is faithful.

(Hebrews 10:23)

CHAPTER FOUR

Matthew

I'm Matthew and this is my story. I was brought up in a non-Christian family but was made to go to Sunday School as a child because that was the 'done' thing for children when I was young. I learned all the Bible stories as a child but stopped going to church when we moved to the north of England when I was 11. I had some kind of relationship with God but it was mostly confined to asking for help when I was desperate to escape the wrath of an angry teacher at school! It was only when I went to Oxford University to study Geology when I was 18 that I started to attend chapel and after many conversations with the University Chaplain I decided I wanted to get serious about God and committed my life to Jesus.

After university I moved to Leeds where I met Adelina, and after two years we got married. As most people do we waited a couple of years after getting married and then felt the time was right to start a family. It never crossed our minds that we would have problems conceiving. Infertility was a big taboo subject, never spoken about amongst friends and certainly not at church. There was no family history of difficulties having children and we were both young so why would there be an issue?

After two unsuccessful years we were referred by our GP to the infertility clinic at our local hospital. But even then we still had problems with our referral letter getting lost which only added to our frustrations.

During these years we became increasingly discouraged, particularly when other couples seemed to have children at the drop of a hat. On one occasion I remember going to visit some friends and their new baby and Adelina was asked if she wanted to hold the baby. I knew that this was the very last thing she wanted to do but she did and I admire how brave she was during those difficult years.

Our consultant recommended IVF, which after a lot of prayer and counsel with close friends we decided to pursue. Thankfully through that we were blessed with our beautiful daughter Hannah!

All through this journey we questioned why we were going through this. What had we done wrong? Were we guilty of any unconfessed sins? If the Bible says, 'Be fruitful and increase in number' (Genesis 1:28) and 'Children are a heritage from the Lord, offspring a reward from him' (Psalm 127:3), then why were we not seeing this truth in our lives? It's reassuring that there are so many stories of infertility in the Bible: you know these problems are on God's radar, he cares about it, and you know it isn't a situation where he is unable to bring hope and fruit.

Going through this has been the biggest challenge to my faith that I've ever faced. When our prayers aren't answered the way we wish you question whether you are praying in accordance with God's will. When the answer is yes, I am praying in accordance with God's will and this still isn't happening, then you wonder whether God is real or even cares? I'd find myself thinking 'they're not even married' or 'they've already got three children, why is God giving them more children?' Jesus said of God the Father: 'He causes his sun to rise on the evil and the good, and sends rain on the righteous and the unrighteous (Matthew 5:45). By this Jesus is meaning that God blesses people regardless of them deserving that blessing because he's a good father and it's his nature to bless and give good gifts.

There's no simple answer to this dilemma of why am I not seeing my prayers being answered how I want. But after years of questioning God the biggest thing I've learned from our situation is not to waste time asking God why but instead to ask him what do you want me to *learn* through this? Through studying the Psalms, we see how David was very real with God. I can't picture David politely praying this:

My God, my God, why have you forsaken me?
  Why are you so far from saving me,
  so far from my cries of anguish?
My God, I cry out by day, but you do not answer,
  by night, but I find no rest.

(Psalm 22:1–2)

He would have been crying out in distress, praying and feeling those same emotions that Adelina and I had been experiencing. I'm usually a typically reserved British man so it's really comforting to know that we can relate to God in this way. One Saturday we sat in our car in the car park of a large shopping centre telling God exactly how we felt. Years of pent up anger and frustration came flooding out. It was hugely cathartic being so honest with each other and God to the extent that we feared getting hit by a heavenly thunderbolt when we got out of the car! We did eventually get out and lived to tell the tale!

For any couples going through infertility my best advice would be to find another couple who have been through the same thing to come alongside you and support you through it. It's very difficult for people who haven't experienced it to know how best to pray and support you and know what to say (and sometimes saying nothing is best). It can even be difficult sharing difficulties with parents and other family members. Knowing that you have permission to be real with God and each other is also equally important. Continuing to worship God is key too. The words to a song by the band Tonex, 'God Has Not Forgot' were really helpful for me. Whatever songs help you, use them to keep you in a place of praise.

PART TWO

Infertility in the Bible

One of the key aspects of me understanding and moving into a position of overcoming for my own infertility journey was discovering what the Bible and God had to say about it. I picked out the Bible's infertility stories so we can grasp the man's point of view and look at the husband's character and see how their examples give us something to learn from and help us 'man up' and be the men and supportive husbands we need to be. I've summed up the key learning points at the end of the chapter. I always think it's good to challenge yourself with some honest questions when you are studying the Bible so I've added a few to each story for you to think about or even discuss with your wife or a trusted friend.

CHAPTER FIVE

Abraham

Genesis 11:27 – Genesis 25:11

The most famous story of overcoming infertility in the Bible is that of Abraham and Sarah. This one's quite a deep one so you might want to make yourself comfy and get yourself a beverage of your choice before diving in! Abraham's story begins at the end of Genesis 11 and start of chapter 12 where God calls the man who was at that point still named Abram to leave his home and family to follow him:

> The LORD had said to Abram, 'Go from your country, your people and your father's household to the land I will show you.
>
> 'I will make you into a great nation,
>   and I will bless you;
> I will make your name great,
>   and you will be a blessing.
> I will bless those who bless you,
>   and whoever curses you I will curse;
> and all peoples on earth
>   will be blessed through you.
>
> *(Genesis 12:1–3)*

In three short verses God promises to make Abraham into a great nation, make his name great, bless him and show a brief outline of his future plan to redeem humanity where 'all' people would be blessed because of him through Jesus! Abraham's part in this covenant with God was simply to obey God and follow him. We need to follow Abraham's example, whether that means uprooting your family and moving to a foreign land or simply to put God first at work, in business, relationships or the simple choices of daily life. All these promises begin with the simple command to 'go'. 'Go' is one of the shortest words in the dictionary but one of the hardest things to do. Before Abraham could walk into his destiny he had to 'go', leaving his own country and family behind to follow God. Whatever we do in life we must be willing to follow God's calling and 'go' wherever he calls us.

All through Genesis Abraham was told by God that he was going to bless him with a family who were going to inherit the land of Caanan. Every time God spoke, more details of the plan were revealed to Abraham: 'To your offspring I will give this land' (Genesis 12:7.

Further promises were given in following chapters:

Look around from where you are, to the north and south, to the east and west. All the land that you see I will give to you and your offspring forever. I will make your offspring like the dust of the earth, so that if anyone could count the dust, then your offspring could be counted. Go, walk through the length and breadth of the land, for I am giving it to you.

(Genesis 13:14–17)

But despite these promises, a child was not given to them immediately, and during this time of waiting, doubts and fears surely began to fill his mind. Life was not straightforward for Abraham either and included problems with his extended family when he and his nephew Lot went their separate ways. Lot chose to live in Sodom and ended up being taken prisoner by a group of kings. Abraham led a group of his men in a night-time assault and rescued Lot, his family and possessions. After the rescue God says: 'Do not be afraid, Abram. I am your shield, your very great reward' (Genesis 15:1).

This is the first time in Scripture where God tells someone not to be afraid! How many times do we still need to hear this message? God is telling Abraham that above all the blessings he is giving to him, *God himself* is his major blessing. It's not the receiving of a child that is the ultimate blessing, nor is it the blessings of wealth or possessions. Instead, God is Abraham's 'shield' and 'very great reward', both greater than any child, no matter how many years they have been longed for. We can miss the blessings that a relationship with God has to offer if we focus on what we can get out of it, especially if our focus is on children or any other material 'thing' that we desire. Our focus should be on the 'Prince' and not the 'prize', the 'Giver' and not the 'gift'. This is a lesson that Abraham ultimately learned, and we see his obedience to God when he is tested and asked to sacrifice his son Isaac in Genesis 22. In a future prophetic glimpse of God the Father sacrificing his own son Jesus, Abraham was willing to sacrifice his 'gift' for the sake of obedience to the 'Giver'. Although Abraham didn't need to sacrifice Isaac in the end because God provided a lamb (as another prophetic image of Jesus), Hebrews tells us that Abraham was willing to do it because he thought God would raise him from death:

> By faith Abraham, when God tested him, offered Isaac as a sacrifice. He who had embraced the promises was about

to sacrifice his one and only son, even though God had said to him, 'It is through Isaac that your offspring will be reckoned.' Abraham reasoned that God could even raise the dead, and so in a manner of speaking he did receive Isaac back from death.

(Hebrews 11:17–19)

What incredible faith Abraham had! God did go that one step further by sending Jesus to be *our* sacrificial lamb two thousand years later and for that we should be eternally grateful.

Before we get ahead of ourselves with the birth of Isaac we need to look at Abraham's situation. The big problem for him was that he was already old. Abraham was 75 years old when he was first called out of Haran and Sarah was around 65, naturally speaking way too old to be having children and whilst it's all well and good receiving promises, you want to start seeing them fulfilled before too long. You can understand why Abraham was feeling impatient with the delay and is almost accusatory in his next exchange with God:

'Sovereign LORD, what can you give me since I remain childless and the one who will inherit my estate is Eliezer of Damascus?' And Abram said, 'You have given me no children; so a servant in my household will be my heir.' Then the word of the LORD came to him: 'This man will not be your heir, but a son who is your own flesh and blood will be your heir.' He took him outside and said, 'Look up at the sky and count the stars – if indeed you can count them.' Then he said to him, 'So shall your offspring be.'

(Genesis 15:2–6)

God confirms that Abraham's heir will be his own son, his own flesh and blood, and not an adopted servant. God takes him out of his tent and shows Abraham all the stars in the sky to show him exactly how many his ancestors will be. Sometimes God has to take you out from where you are before he can show you how much he can do. When we're all doom and gloom and feeling down you lose sight of how big God is and how much He can do in your life. Taking time out maybe for a weekend retreat, some time in the country side or whatever works for you can take you out of your present situation into the reality of all that God can do. This encounter with God clearly had a dramatic effect on Abraham because in the next verse we are told, 'Abram believed the LORD, and he credited it to him as righteousness' (Genesis 15:6).

Whilst Abraham had been told that he would have his own 'flesh and blood' family, God had so far said nothing about Sarah being the mother. As the years passed since that first promise (around ten or eleven years as we are told Abraham was 86 when Ishmael was born), Sarah took matters into her own hands and in Genesis 16 we are told the story of Hagar and the birth of Ishmael. Whilst seeming highly unorthodox to our times, the custom of taking a slave girl to produce an heir was a practised custom thousands of years ago. Cuneiform clay tablets found by archaeologists describe the custom of an infertile wife choosing a slave to have a child with her husband; the child would then 'belong' to the wife and be the legal heir. Sarah said to Abraham:

> The LORD has kept me from having children. Go, sleep with my slave; perhaps I can build a family through her. Abram agreed to what Sarai said. So after Abram had been living in Canaan ten years, Sarai his wife took her Egyptian slave Hagar and gave her to her husband to be his wife. He slept with Hagar, and she conceived. When she knew she was pregnant, she began to despise her mistress.
>
> *(Genesis 16:2–4)*

How often do we get inpatient with God when things don't work out the way we planned, and instead of continually trusting him we try to force things through, with the results being messy and disastrous. This is the case here too as Sarah's plan for Abraham to have a child with her slave Hagar ends in bitterness between the women, and ultimately Abraham has to send Hagar and his son Ishmael away after Isaac was born, a decision that must have been very difficult for Abraham. Even though Ishmael (meaning 'God hears') was not the child promised by God, he was still faithful to Abraham and chose to make him into a great nation (Genesis 17:20).

We can think of Bible characters as being incredibly holy but as we have just seen with Hagar, throughout his life Abraham made mistakes, even making the same one twice by not trusting God to protect him and lying about Sarah not being his wife. Still God remained faithful to him and when we make mistakes in our battle with infertility God is always merciful and forgives us too:

> Because of the LORD's great love we are not consumed, for his compassions never fail. They are new every morning; great is your faithfulness.
>
> *(Lamentations 3:22–23)*

Even when we doubt, get angry, feel jealous or even give up on him, God is always merciful. What an incredible God!

I know that I probably don't need to include this next part but I will anyway. Most people would never consider this, but if you're a man reading this don't even think of having a child with someone not your wife (or indeed a woman reading this with another man). Don't even entertain those thoughts in your mind because that's the first step towards that sin. It's only going to end in pain for you, your wife, the 'other' woman and any children you have. It's never God's way and this is not an option for you in the battle with infertility. It's just a scheme of the Enemy (the devil) to deceive you. Look at Abraham's example and learn from it. The results were jealousy, anger and a broken family unit. Of course, God can bring good out of any situation, and I've seen first-hand an amazing example of how a child born out of an affair can become loved and accepted by the whole family, but this is not how God intends things to be.

When Abraham was ninety-nine God spoke to him again:

'. . . I am God Almighty; walk before me faithfully and be blameless. Then I will make my covenant between me and you and will greatly increase your numbers.'

Abram fell facedown, and God said to him, 'As for me, this is my covenant with you: You will be the father of many nations. No longer will you be called Abram; your name will be Abraham, for I have made you a father of many nations. I will make you very fruitful; I will make nations of you, and kings will come from you. I will establish my covenant as an everlasting covenant between me and you and your descendants after you for the generations to come, to be your God and the God of your descendants after you. The whole land of Canaan, where you now reside as a foreigner, I will give as an everlasting possession to you and your descendants after you; and I will be their God.'

(Genesis 17:1–8)

In a highly important gesture, God changes Abram's name from 'exalted father' to Abraham, 'father of multitudes'. God adds an 'h' to Abraham's name (the original spelling of Abram is actually Abraam) and this 'h' symbolises the life-giving 'breath of God'. I don't want to get too technical but I think it's important to explain this a bit deeper. God's name in Hebrew is YHWH (pronounced Yahweh in English as there are no vowels written in Hebrew) and adding the 'h' from YHWH that symbolises God's spirit and breath is so significant. It's like God is adding his spirit, breath and a part of his name to Abraham. It's the same powerful 'breath' that spoke the world into creation, breathed life into Adam's nostrils and was able to create life again, this time for Abraham and Sarah. Also Sarai's name, meaning 'princess', was also changed to Sarah with the addition of another 'h', meaning 'mother of nations', and for the first time God reveals that Sarah is going to be the mother of Abraham's promised child.

'As for Sarai your wife, you are no longer to call her Sarai; her name will be Sarah. I will bless her and will surely give you a son by her. I will bless her so that she will be the mother of nations; kings of peoples will come from her.

(Genesis 17:15–16)

Whenever God changed peoples' names in the Bible it was to confirm a new identity. Jacob, whose name meant 'supplanter', becoming Israel, which means 'having power with God' (Genesis 32:28) and Simon – 'God has heard' – became Peter – 'rock'(Matthew 16 v 17-18). For Abraham and Sarah, their new identity would be father and mother of multitudes and of nations. The very act of changing and then speaking out each other's names would serve to remind them of God's promise and be an act of faith as they were seemingly as far away as ever from seeing a child. Abraham was unable to hide his disbelief with God:

Abraham fell face down; he laughed and said to himself, 'Will a son be born to a man a hundred years old? Will

Sarah bear a child at the age of ninety?' And Abraham said to God, 'If only Ishmael might live under your blessing!'

(Genesis 17:17–18)

Despite meeting with God and having the promises reaffirmed, Abraham still didn't believe God and laughed when he told him Sarah would have a baby. In the same way, it's hard for us to keep trusting God when our circumstances don't correspond to what his Word says. Abraham showed his doubts by again suggesting that God should fulfil his covenant through Ishmael, but God's ways were better.

In the next chapter, Genesis 18, Abraham is told by one of God's messengers on their way to destroy Sodom and Gomorrah that, 'I will surely return to you about this time next year, and Sarah your wife will have a son.' (verse 10).

Sarah was listening to this exchange at the tent door. We don't know why she wasn't with Abraham at the time when he was meeting with the messenger. Maybe it was cultural or maybe all their shared disappointments were putting their relationship under strain. No marriage is immune to difficulties and going through the fire of infertility will leave couples under enormous stress. It's especially important for husbands (and wives) to recognise this potential problem and take steps to maintain the relationship and protect the partnership so we can face God together.

So Sarah laughed to herself as she thought, 'After I am worn out and my lord is old, will I now have this pleasure?'

Then the LORD said to Abraham, 'Why did Sarah laugh and say, "Will I really have a child, now that I am old?" Is anything too hard for the LORD? I will return to you at the appointed time next year, and Sarah will have a son.'

(Genesis 18:12–15)

Like Abraham, Sarah's response to God's promise was laughter. Our faith needs to be in God and not our circumstances. Jesus told this to his disappointed and dejected disciples after they had unsuccessfully tried to heal a boy with epilepsy: 'Truly I tell you, if you have faith as small as a mustard seed, you can say to this mountain, "Move from here to there," and it will move. Nothing will be impossible for you' (Matthew 17:20).

The 'mountain' in your life may be infertility or it may be some other kind of sickness or problem that may seem like an insurmountable object, but when we are full of faith we see God standing behind that mountain just waiting to move it for us.

In the next chapter, Genesis 19, we read the story of the destruction of Sodom and Gomorrah and the escape of Lot and his family. Lot's wife dies and Lot and his daughters flee and live alone in a cave. Lot's daughters feared that they wouldn't have children so came up with a plan to get their father drunk and sleep with him to get pregnant. Their plan was successful and the older daughter had a son named Moab and the younger daughter also had a son and she named him Ben-Ammi. (Genesis 19 v 31-38). Quite what Abraham must have thought of this we don't know. If it was me, I'd have been furious about the situation. Abraham had played a part in saving Lot and his family from the destruction of Sodom and Gomorrah (Genesis 19:29) and now Lot's two daughters had become pregnant by their father. Looking on from the outside you could say that it looks like they had been rewarded for their sinful behaviour and received a blessing that Abraham was desperately hoping and trusting God for. You might find yourself feeling similar feelings of anger, jealousy and a sense of injustice when other people have children after a 'one-night' stand, the result of an affair or when people seem to get pregnant very easily. It doesn't seem fair and makes us question God. All we can do in these situations is to keep on trusting God and avoid falling into bitterness and anger. Both of the sons born to Lot's daughters became the ancestors of the Moabites and Ammonites, people who ended up the enemies of Abraham's offspring for centuries, which only highlights further the long-term implications of sin.

Just before Isaac was born there was another fascinating episode in the life of Abraham, found in Genesis 20, where he and Sarah go to live in Gerar. Abraham must have been afraid of the king of Gerar, Abimelek, and so he told Sarah to say that she was his sister. Because of this lie Abimelek takes Sarah into his household. Before Abimelek can sleep with her God warns him in a dream to return Sarah to Abraham otherwise he and his household will die. In addition God stops Abimelek's wife and female slaves from becoming pregnant. Abraham after being confronted by Abimelek prayed for healing and Abimelek's wife and slaves were healed from their temporary infertility:

> Then Abraham prayed to God, and God healed Abimelek, his wife and his female slaves so they could have children again, for the LORD had kept all the women in Abimelek's household from conceiving because of Abraham's wife Sarah.
>
> *(Genesis 20:17–18)*

Just as in the story of Lot's daughters getting pregnant, the Bible doesn't tell us how Abraham felt about this but you can imagine seeing a successful infertility healing for a pagan king and his household could have been demoralising. I was Abraham I'd have been asking God,

'How could you heal these godless Philistines when my own wife remains barren?'

Instead Abraham obediently prays and the result is the first recorded healing in Scripture. I think through this we should learn that even though our own hearts are grieving through infertility we should still be faithfully praying for others to conceive too. One time I was in church and the pastor asked if anyone had a word from God to share. In my heart I felt relieved that I didn't, but then as soon I thought that, God told me to go to the front and pray for people struggling to have children. I felt so angry and humiliated that God wanted me to stand at the front of church and pray, knowing full well that lots of people in church knew our circumstances. I was trying to hold back the tears but knew God desires obedience, so I did what he asked and I prayed for a girl who bravely came forwards for prayer. Years later she did in fact have a much hoped for child! We've prayed with many couples to have children and in most cases they have gone on to have families. I'm not going to lie, it's not easy seeing them receive the blessing that we have been praying for, but we want good things for our friends and want to 'rejoice' with them. I've found that sharing other people's joy is the perfect antidote to the bitterness that could so easily consume my heart. Maybe this miracle of Abimalek's household being healed from their infertility strengthened Abraham's faith, that if God could do it for a pagan king, surely he could do the same for me too?

It's in Genesis 21:1–7 that we finally see the promise fulfilled, 25 years after God first called him out of Haran, with the birth of Isaac (which means 'laughter', showing Abraham and Sarah's sense of humour because they both laughed when God told them they were going to have a child!). Paul, writing in Romans thousands of years later, says of Abraham:

> Against all hope, Abraham in hope believed and so became the father of many nations, just as it had been said to him, 'So shall your offspring be.' Without weakening in his faith, he faced the fact that his body was as good as dead – since he was about a hundred years old – and that Sarah's

womb was also dead. Yet he did not waver through unbelief regarding the promise of God, but was strengthened in his faith and gave glory to God, being fully persuaded that God had power to do what he had promised.

(Romans 4:18–21)

What an amazing legacy to leave. That even though he considered his own body to be dead he still knew God was able to fulfil his promises. Whatever circumstances we might be facing in our lives, be that infertility or any other problems like sickness, debt, depression, we have a God we serve who can do all things. God had kept his promises to Abraham and Sarah and he will keep his promises to you too!

'Jesus Christ is the same yesterday and today and forever.'

Hebrews 13 v 8

Lessons from Abraham
- Abraham was obedient to God's call to 'go'.
- Nothing is impossible for God.
- God himself is the real prize, not the baby.
- God keeps his promises whilst we need to stay obedient.
- Don't do things in your own strength.
- God's timing is perfect.
- God always has the bigger picture in mind.
- Pray for others going through infertility.

Questions
- How can we keep trusting God when things don't work out how we'd like?

- Where is God calling me to 'go'?
- What areas of our lives do we try to take matters into our own hands instead of trusting in God?
- Do my circumstances make me doubt the truth of God's Word?
- How can we support other people battling infertility?
- How do I feel when people around me are blessed with a family and I'm not?

CHAPTER SIX

Isaac

Genesis 25:19 – 26

Isaac as we've just read was the miracle son of Abraham and Sarah. He would have been well aware of the circumstances of his birth and the inheritance God had promised to his father. In some respects, we may be surprised that Isaac suffered in the same way as his father, but equally the Enemy would have been keen to try to cut off the line of God's future Messiah, Jesus.

Genesis 25 tells us that Isaac was 40 when he married Rebekah and 60 when his twin sons Jacob and Esau were born. That's 20 years of waiting for a promise to be fulfilled! In our world of instant gratification, waiting five minutes in a queue seems like a lifetime! We waited seven years for the blessing of our adopted family and that was an incredibly frustrating time, so the thought of waiting 20 years for a family seems hard to contemplate. It wouldn't have been uncommon for a man in those days to take more than one wife and so it's to Isaac's credit that he chose not to and demonstrated his love and loyalty to Rebekah. The Bible doesn't say but it could also have simply been wisdom from Isaac that stopped him from choosing another wife and showed that he had learned from his father's mistakes with

Hagar and Ishamael. It's certainly better and less painful to learn from other's mistakes than learning a lesson the hard way.

So what else can we learn from Isaac? The Bible only tells us a few details about Isaac and Rebekah's journey but what it does tell us is hugely significant: 'Isaac prayed to the LORD on behalf of his wife, because she was childless. The LORD answered his prayer, and his wife Rebekah became pregnant' (Genesis 25:21).

Prayer must always be our first response to facing infertility. We can get blasé about praying but I don't think we realise the power we have in our hands. When we pray we're communicating with the creator of the whole universe! As followers of Jesus we are to 'Rejoice always, pray continually, give thanks in all circumstances; for this is God's will for you in Christ Jesus' (1 Thessalonians 5:16–18).

These things are far from easy but by always rejoicing, praying and being thankful our lives will be much more fruitful and will stop the depression, anxiety and disappointment that comes with facing infertility.

In the Sermon on the Mount Jesus tells us this:

Ask and it will be given to you; seek and you will find; knock and the door will be opened to you. For everyone who asks receives; the one who seeks finds; and to the one who knocks, the door will be opened.

(Matthew 7:7–8)

Some translations even add 'keep on asking', suggesting that our prayers aren't always answered instantaneously in the way we want. Jesus isn't saying that whatever we ask for we'll get – so don't bother asking to win the lottery – but rather if we ask for good things in line with his will then we will receive what we need. We know that if we ask for families without selfish thoughts this is in line with God's will.

I think it's interesting that Genesis says Isaac prayed 'on behalf' of his wife. Sometimes your wife may be struggling so much you may have to pray 'on behalf' of her like just Isaac did. At other times you may be the one struggling, so your wife may be the one praying. This is what often happened in our situation. The point is, you need to be there for each other and at certain times, when the other partner is struggling, you may need to pray for them. We know God always hears our prayers and is consistently a good father and this is seen with the blessing of twin sons Jacob and Esau (Genesis 25 v 24-26).

Lessons from Isaac

- Isaac stayed faithful to God even though it took years to see a breakthrough.
- Isaac remained loyal to his wife when he could have taken other wives.
- Learned from his father's mistakes. It's better to learn from other's mistakes than make them ourselves.
- Isaac prayed on behalf of his wife.

Questions

- Am I praying consistently?
- What specific mistakes have people made in this book? What can I do to avoid making them?
- Am I misunderstanding God's Word? In what ways?
- Are my prayers in line with God's will for my life?

CHAPTER SEVEN

Jacob

Genesis 29:31 – Genesis 35:20

Jacob, along with his twin brother Esau, was the much longed for son of Isaac and Rebekah. There's a lot we can learn from this story about family and sibling rivalries. With the help of his mother Rebekah, Jacob tricked his brother out of his birth right as the oldest son then fled to escape Esau's wrath. Jacob went to Haran and worked for his uncle Laban taking care of his goats. Laban had two daughters, Leah the elder sister and Rachel. Rachel was beautiful and Jacob fell madly in love with her and agreed to work seven years in return for marrying her. When the time came for the marriage Laban tricked Jacob into marrying Leah because she was the older sister (the custom of the time was that the eldest sister had to marry first). When Jacob discovered the deception, he confronted Laban and was allowed to marry Rachel in return for another seven years of work. Whatever family circumstances you find yourself in it's reassuring to read that families in the Bible weren't all perfect and God understands the complexities of family dynamics. I hope you've followed that because it's about to get even more strange!

Genesis 29:30 tells us that Jacob loved Rachel more than her sister, but despite this Leah was blessed with children whilst

Rachel remained barren: 'When the LORD saw that Leah was not loved, he enabled her to conceive, but Rachel remained childless' (Genesis 29:31). Leah initially went onto have four sons whilst Rachel had none.

The situation lead to jealousy between the two sisters and started a bitter family feud. Jealousy and envy are common emotions amongst couples facing infertility but if left to fester they can lead to further emotions of anger, depression and the breakdown of relationships, even among family members. The apostle James puts it like this: 'For where you have envy and selfish ambition, there you find disorder and every evil practice' (James 3:16).

The jealousy between Rebekah and Leah led to a strange situation where Jacob ended up having children with both wives' slaves in some kind of bizarre baby competition (Genesis 30 v 3-12)! While this was the custom during that time, you wouldn't believe this kind of story would feature in a television soap opera let alone be found in the Bible! As the tension simmered between the sisters, sons were being born who would become the twelve tribes of Israel, so even through all this chaos God was still working to achieve his purposes.

At the start of Genesis 30 we read of Rachel's anguish at not being able to have a family: 'When Rachel saw that she was not bearing Jacob any children, she became jealous of her sister. So she said to Jacob, "Give me children, or I'll die!"' (verse 1).

Whilst the thought of dying because you can't have children does sound extreme to people on the outside, for those going through the monthly agony of a negative pregnancy test it rings true. If you ever find yourself going down this thought path STOP and talk to someone!

If you ever feel that having a family is the most important thing in your life it's a warning sign that your priorities aren't in the right order. In this instance, for Rachel, the *gift* had assumed greater importance than the one who gives the gift. The desire to have children, although a completely natural and godly feeling, can be used by the Enemy, and if we take our eyes off Jesus and our goal becomes the *gift* rather than *giver* we are in danger of making the gift of children into a false idol in our lives. Jesus tells us in Matthew 6 to 'seek first his kingdom and his righteousness, and all these things will be given to you as well (verse 33).

I often pray this prayer over my wife and I to remind us that our 'first' priority is to seek God's kingdom; we need to focus on Jesus at all times. If we start off on the right foot by seeking Jesus above all else, we cannot go wrong.

Personally, one of the most painful things about our infertility journey was seeing how upset my wife got every month when things hadn't work out as we'd hoped. I was constantly amazed at how soon she bounced back, full of faith for the next month, but I think being a woman and being the one who is 'not pregnant' is a burden and pressure we men don't face and perhaps one we don't understand as well as we might. Naturally, the monthly disappointment is a difficult time for both husband and wife but Jacob, in his frustration with the situation was getting angry with his wife and God: 'Jacob became angry with her and said, "Am I in the place of God, who has kept you from having children?"' (Genesis 30:2)

We all get angry from time to time, but anger is never a good way to answer your wife's distress no matter how difficult you might be finding it yourself, and it's not going to help the situation. Being real and honest with God when you're feeling rubbish and annoyed is completely OK and what God wants to hear from us as our best friend. David, throughout the Psalms, expressed his doubts, fears and frustrations with God many times and we too can be confident he will hear us. Paul puts it like this,

"In your anger do not sin": Do not let the sun go down while you are still angry, and do not give the devil a foothold." Ephesians 4 v 26-27.

Anger in itself is not sinful but it can certainly lead to sin. Allowing anger into your life and marriage does give the devil a foothold to cause pain so be very careful with this emotion. Blaming God for our difficulties is not the answer either. We know that God is good all the time but we *don't* and *can't* understand his ways all the time. Paul states this in Romans 11:

> Oh, the depth of the riches of the wisdom and
> knowledge of God!
> How unsearchable his judgments,
> and his paths beyond tracing out!
> 'Who has known the mind of the Lord?
> Or who has been his counsellor?'
>
> *(Romans 11:33–34)*

All we can do is trust and keep on trusting him. There's no good answer to the 'Why us, God?' question. When God created the world in Genesis 1 he declared it 'very good'. Since sin came into the world in the Garden of Eden as the consequences of Adam and Eve's wrong choices the results have been sickness (including infertility and miscarriage) and death. We can't understand why some people experience infertility and others don't but God has provided us with the ultimate answer to life's struggles in his son Jesus! One of the clearest prophecies of Jesus is found in Isaiah 53:

> Surely he took up our pain
> and bore our suffering,
> yet we considered him punished by God,
> stricken by him, and afflicted.

But he was pierced for our transgressions,
    he was crushed for our iniquities;
the punishment that brought us peace was on him,
    and by his wounds we are healed.

(Isaiah 53:4–5)

When Jesus died on the cross he died for both our salvation *and* our healing. That healing power is still freely available to us all, but why some people get to see healing from their infertility and others don't is an incredibly difficult question. My answer is that infertility was never part of God's original plan for creation, and we must keep on trusting and expecting God to do a healing miracle. Like those three brave friends who faced the fiery furnace, I'm going to trust that God can deliver us – and even if he doesn't I'm still going to keep on trusting!

Eventually, God heard Rachel's prayers:

Then God remembered Rachel; he listened to her and enabled her to conceive. She became pregnant and gave birth to a son and said, 'God has taken away my disgrace.' She named him Joseph, and said, 'May the Lord add to me another son.'

(Genesis 30:22–24)

Joseph goes on to follow in the footsteps of Isaac and Jacob and becomes the third-generation man to be born after infertility. This pattern keeps repeating itself in Scripture where significant men of God are born to couples who have struggled to conceive. It's important to remember that ultimately it is God who 'enables' us to have children and not doctors or medicine. The moment we take our eyes off God and look to medicine as the source of healing can lead to trouble.

Lessons from Jacob

- Family dynamics are complicated and sometimes messy. God understands this.
- Don't get angry with your wife or God.
- In your anger do not sin.
- Don't allow jealousy to affect your relationships with family and friends.
- God answers the prayers for children consistently over three generations.

Questions

- Do I blame God for infertility?
- Do I get angry at my wife or God because of infertility?
- Is having children of greater importance in my life than my relationship with God?
- How is infertility affecting my relationships with family and friends?
- Are these relationships stronger or are they adversely affected?
- What do I need to do to improve these relationships?

CHAPTER EIGHT

Manoah

Judges 13 – 16

The story of the circumstances leading up to the birth of Samson is one of the most remarkable in the Bible but least known. Starting in Judges 13, we read that the Israelites had once again rebelled against God and were in a period of 40 years of domination by the Philistines. It is during this time of rebellion that we learn about Samson's father Manoah (meaning place of rest) and his unnamed wife. Judges doesn't tell us how long they had been without children but presumably it was a significant amount of time because Manoah's wife was known as barren. Judges 13 tells us:

A certain man of Zorah, named Manoah, from the clan of the Danites, had a wife who was childless, unable to give birth. The angel of the Lord appeared to her and said, 'You are barren and childless, but you are going to become pregnant and give birth to a son. Now see to it that you drink no wine or other fermented drink and that you do not eat anything unclean. You will become pregnant and have a son whose head is never to be touched by a razor because the boy is to be a Nazirite, dedicated to God from the womb. He will take the lead in delivering Israel from the hands of the Philistines.'

(Judges 13:2–5)

Just as the Israelites were crying out for a saviour to deliver them from the Philistines, God sends them one. The parallels with Jesus are striking, where an angel is sent to a seemingly insignificant woman to tell her she's going to have a miracle baby son who was sent by God to deliver his people. Manoah's wife went and told her husband all the words of the angel. This strong relationship between husband and wife is vitally important; Manoah's wife shared her experience of the angel visiting her and he was greatly encouraged. Marriage is a partnership and sharing encouraging words and our personal experiences of God is really important to maintaining a strong marriage through hard times. However, before we do this, we need to make sure that we are regularly spending time with God, reading and listening to his Word, to receive our own personal encouragement. At difficult times this can feel like the last thing we want to do but it is essential to maintaining a good relationship with God.

When Manoah heard about the angel's words he doesn't question them but instantly believes. I don't know about you, but if my wife told me an angel had visited her, my first question would be have you been drinking and if so how much! Not only does Manoah have the faith to believe he will have a son, he recognises how incredibly blessed he is and that his son is going to be a special child. Because of this Manoah immediately asks God for help in bringing up his son: 'Pardon your servant, Lord. I beg you to let the man of God you sent to us come again to teach us how to bring up the boy who is to be born' (Judges 13:8).

Manoah wanted to make sure he did his best as a father so that Samson would fulfil his potential and be prepared for the work God had for him. All children are special but in the Bible the children of parents who have battled through infertility were used massively by God. The Enemy knows our potential and the potential of our children and certainly doesn't want them to be born. So even though we may not have children yet we should be asking God for help in bringing them up just as Manoah did so that when that day comes we're ready to be the best fathers we can be! As Proverbs tells us: 'Start children off on the way they should go, and even when they are old they will not turn from it' (Proverbs 22:6).

God's angel revisits Manoah and his wife and reminds them of his commands to bring their son up as a Nazirite (someone dedicated to God). Afterwards Manoah offers a sacrifice to God to give thanks for the blessing that he is about to receive. It's always good to give thanks for all the blessings that God gives us, but particularly to give thanks in advance. Rick Warren, American pastor and author, says, 'Faith is thanking God in advance', and this is exactly what Manoah does.

In fact, it is the faith of Manoah that impresses me the most about this man. Three times he shows his faith, firstly by not questioning the words of the angel when he hears that he will have a son, and twice when he says to the angel, 'when your words come true' in Judges 13:12 and 17 (emphasis my own). When God promises you something that word is true. As it says in Numbers 23: 'God is not human, that he should lie, not a human being, that he should change his mind. Does he speak and then not act? Does he promise and not fulfil?' (verse 19). Jesus himself said 'your word is truth' (John 17:17).

Faith in God and his word is a key element to this battle with infertility and we can have total confidence in God's truth. Truth always beats facts.

Judges 13 ends with the birth of Samson, a man blessed by God and directed by the spirit of God. In some translations of the Bible, we are told that the angel said he will 'begin' to save Israel from the Philistines (verse 5). Maybe his potential was to totally save Israel, but by his foolish acts he almost loses everything. God never forgot him though and Samson's life, whilst looking like a failure, ends in his redemption as the temple of the Philistines comes crashing down under Samson's God-given strength. Maybe this is how you're feeling now? Infertility or some other problem makes you feel like a failure but this is not the end of your story and whilst there's still breath in your body God can redeem any situation.

One final point we can learn from this story is found after Samson's death where we learn that Samson had brothers: 'Then his brothers and his father's whole family went down to get him. They brought him back and buried him between Zorah and Eshtaol in the tomb of Manoah his father' (Judges 16:31). God had clearly blessed Manoah and his wife with a family that was much more than they could have believed, and he can do the same for you too!

> Now to him who is able to do immeasurably more than all we ask or imagine, according to his power that is at work within us, to him be glory in the church and in Christ Jesus throughout all generations, forever and ever! Amen.
>
> *(Ephesians 3:20–21)*

God has shown that he has his own timing, not ours. His timing is incredibly hard to fathom but we know God has good plans for us, and just as in this story God had a plan for Samson, he has good plans for you too whatever your future may hold.

Lessons from Manoah

- A strong relationship with your wife is important, as is sharing your experiences of God.
- We must believe and not question God's word.
- We can speak to God just like we would to a friend.
- God can help us know how to bring up our children, even before they are born or adopted.
- Recognised his responsibility in bringing up his son.
- In faith gave thanks before receiving the blessing.
- We can receive blessings beyond what we expect and hope for.

Questions

- When God tells me something do I instantly believe it?
- Am I praying for my unborn children?
- How am I encouraging my spouse in this journey?
- Do I believe God's promises? If not, what is preventing me from believing?

CHAPTER NINE

Elkanah

1 Samuel 1:1 – 1 Samuel 2:21

Hannah's husband is the forgotten half of one of the most famous Bible stories of overcoming infertility. You probably know the story of Hannah but I bet you can't remember her husband's name! In 1 Samuel 1 we read that Elkanah was from Ephraim, a place which means 'fruitful' or even 'doubly fruitful'. We know he had two wives, Hannah, who was barren, and Peninnah, who had sons and daughters.

In 1 Samual 1:5 it says that God actually kept Hannah from conceiving and 'closed her womb'. I'm not sure why God would do that but we do know that God is omnipotent and beyond our understanding: 'As the heavens are higher than the earth, so are my ways higher than your ways and my thoughts than your thoughts' (Isaiah 55:9).

Trusting in God's timings whilst waiting for a family is difficult but we can be assured that he knows what's best for us and can use delay for some greater purpose: '"For I know the plans I have for you," declares the LORD, "plans to prosper you and not to harm you, plans to give you hope and a future"' (Jeremiah 29:11). I believe part of God's plan in Elkanah and Hannah's story was that we could read this story thousands of years later and be encouraged that he is faithful.

As a husband, a massive part of the infertility battle is supporting our wives as we go through it together. Elkanah was a good man who followed God and made sacrifices every year at Shiloh where the tabernacle and Ark of the Covenant were kept. He would give portions of the sacrificial meat to Peninnah and her children but he showed special affection for Hannah by giving her a double portion of the meat to show that he loved her in spite of her lack of children.

Isaiah also talks about receiving a double portion of blessing: 'Instead of your shame you will receive a double portion, and instead of disgrace you will rejoice in your inheritance. And so you will inherit a double portion in your land, and everlasting joy will be yours' (Isaiah 61:7).

Husbands, take note, Elkanah was showing his wife special love. I don't know many women who wouldn't appreciate special affection, and even more so those struggling with infertility, so however you like to treat your wife, be it gifts, weekend breaks, flowers or even an extra steak like Elkanah, just do it! I'm not great at this, as my wife will no doubt confirm, but we as husbands should make more effort to prioritise quality time with our wives. As a little tip there's a great book by Gary Chapman called The Five Love Languages which helps you understand how your wife receives love. It's too much to go into here but in the book the author describes five love languages- receiving gifts, quality time, words of affirmation, acts of service and physical touch. Everyone has a preference for one or two of these. There's also an online questionnaire to help you understand your wife's key love languages so you can show her love in the ways she will receive best.

1 Samuel 1:7 tells us that 'year after year' Peninnah teased Hannah so much that she wept and stopped eating. As a man and protector Elkanah shouldn't have allowed this in his house and should have 'manned up' and put a stop to it when it first

started. It's unlikely that people would be so cruel as to make fun of you or your wife's misery but as a man and husband you've got to be aware of your wife's emotions and be ready to protect her from gossip.

As men we are not necessarily known for being especially sensitive or observant, two things Elkanah definitely isn't when he asks Hannah, 'Hannah, why are you weeping? Why don't you eat? Why are you downhearted? Don't I mean more to you than ten sons?' 1 (Samuel 1:8).

People are always going to say insensitive things to couples who are struggling to conceive, most often by accident (or ignorance!). It's really upsetting at the time and you need to keep calm and give people a lot of grace. Elkanah's careless words may have been particularly wounding to Hannah because it would have been blatantly obvious why she was so upset; what she needed at her time of distress was comfort. Whilst I'm sure our wives are very grateful to be married to hunks like us, Elkanah's comment that he is worth more than ten sons was maybe not the most sensitive thing to say to an already distraught Hannah!

Hannah's famous prayer for a son and promise to dedicate him to God has inspired countless couples over the years:

In her deep anguish Hannah prayed to the LORD, weeping bitterly. And she made a vow, saying, 'LORD Almighty, if you will only look on your servant's misery and remember me, and not forget your servant but give her a son, then I will give him to the LORD for all the days of his life, and no razor will ever be used on his head.'

(1 Samuel 1:10–11)

Hannah must have looked so desperate that Eli the High Priest thought she had been drinking alcohol. Hannah explained that she had been 'pouring' her heart out to God and then she and Elkanah 'arose and worshipped before the LORD and then went back to their home at Ramah' 1 Samuel 1:19).

Through this battle remember you and your wife are a team, one flesh, one single unit moulded together by God. Our friends the Smiths refer to themselves as 'Team Smith' and it's a great reminder to us that we are part of a team. Staying strong and making time to come together and worship God is a powerful statement of intent and key to overcoming.

It's interesting that this is the only story of infertility in the Bible that mentions the actual act of 'baby making': 'Elkanah made love to his wife Hannah' (1 Samuel 1:19). I don't need to dwell on this too long, but in the midst of fertility kits, body temperatures, correct timings etc. it's all too easy to forget that we're making love rather than it being all about making a baby. Extra sex is definitely one advantage that infertility brings for a man but that doesn't mean it's always easy. In the words of Rodney Trotter in the BBC sitcom Only Fools and Horses: 'I'm at it like a rattlesnake! It's horrible! Some people dream of singing La Traviata at the Royal Opera House, but they don't wanna sing it three times a night.'

God loves sex and created it for our enjoyment. Within the security of marriage it strengthens couples, but the Enemy can use the stress of infertility to rob us of enjoying sex; instead it can lead to tension between husband and wife. If your sexual relationship is becoming difficult it is important that you respect each other in this area, try and keep talking about it, spend time doing things you enjoy together and find ways to reconnect. Sometimes it can become a more significant issue and develop into a deeper emotional and physical problem for example some men may struggle with getting an erection due to the stress of infertility and low mood can cause loss of your sex drive. If you find yourself in this situation don't be embarrassed to seek help as you GP can provide referrals onto therapies that help couples in this area.

Waiting, like Elkanah and Hannah did, just as Abraham had and countless others have since, is never easy. But 'in the course of time Hannah became pregnant and gave birth to a son. She named him Samuel, saying, "Because I asked the LORD for him"' (1 Samuel v 20). Hannah, true to her promise, dedicated Samuel to God and he was brought up in the temple, serving under Eli the priest. Ultimately, he became a mighty man of God, prophet and leader of the nation of Israel. God's timing is always perfect but we often only see that retrospectively. When we finally adopted our first daughter she came to us days after I finished my final medical consultant exams, and looking back there is no way I could or would have studied as hard as I needed to do to pass those exams with a child.

Our story of Elkanah and Hannah ends in 1 Samuel 2. It says that each year they would visit Samuel at the time of the annual offering:

Eli would bless Elkanah and his wife, saying, 'May the Lord give you children by this woman to take the place of the one she prayed for and gave to the Lord.' Then they would go home. And the Lord was gracious to Hannah; she gave birth to three sons and two daughters. Meanwhile, the boy Samuel grew up in the presence of the Lord.

(1 Samuel 2:20–21)

From having no children, Elkanah and Hannah ended up being blessed with six children. That's the character of God – he loves to bless us abundantly!

Lessons from Elkanah

- Showed special love to his wife.
- Don't say anything stupid!
- Make 'love' not 'a baby'.
- Make time to worship God with your spouse.
- God wants to bless us abundantly.

Discussion questions

- How can we protect our wives and ourselves from gossip and malicious talk?
- How can we show special love to our spouses? https://www.5lovelanguages.com/quizzes/
- Do my careless words bring sadness to my spouse? How can I rectify this?
- What examples of God's perfect timing have I seen in my own life?

CHAPTER TEN

The Shunammite Man

2 Kings 4:8–37

Take a moment and try to think what it would be like to wait years for a child and then when they finally come along they die at a young age. Every parent's worst fear happened to this couple, whose story we read about in 2 Kings 4:8–37. The Bible doesn't even tell us their names; instead the wife is simply known as the Shunammite woman, which means she was a native or inhabitant of the town of Shunem, north of Mount Gilboa in ancient Palestine. We know they were a prominent and wealthy couple who became friends of the prophet Elisha and used their wealth to bless him by building him a room to stay in when he visited their home.

One day, Elisha says to the woman through his servant Gehazi: 'You have gone to all this trouble for us. Now what can be done for you?' (2 Kings 4:13). When she responds, I think it's really telling that she doesn't ask for the one thing that she most desperately wanted. Maybe she was too ashamed to even approach the subject, despite it being painfully obvious to everyone around. Going through infertility can be a terribly lonely experience. Like this couple, you may have many material blessings but the one thing that money can't buy is a family. People going through infertility experience complicated feelings of shame, guilt, fear, anger, jealousy and depression, feelings that are incredibly hard to share with family or close friends. We found it really hard to share how we were feeling because people often don't know how to respond and they feel awkward or worry about saying the wrong thing. It certainly affected some friendships albeit strengthening other ones. I think women probably find it easier to share their feelings with other women, but for us men, who don't often talk about 'our feelings', to start opening up about our struggle with infertility is a real challenge. I think one of the problems is that sharing about infertility can make us feel like so much less of a man and no-one wants to feel like that.

The Bible is full of stories of strong friendships between men. David and Jonathan, Shadrach, Meshach and Abednego, Jesus and his disciples, and Paul and Barnabas are all examples. God's blessed me with strong friendships where I've been able to be honest and talk about our situation and how I'm feeling. I'm really grateful for those relationships, but strong friendships don't just happen, they take time and effort over months and years. Part of the Enemy's strategy is to divide and conquer. The last thing you feel like doing when things aren't going well in the battle is to meet up with other people but we're warned about, 'not giving up meeting together, as some are in the habit of doing, but encouraging one another – and all the more as you see the Day approaching.' Hebrews 10:25

Whenever we don't feel like meeting friends we need to 'man up' because we're better and stronger together. Iron has to actually connect with more iron before both of them can be sharpened after all (Proverbs 27 v 17)! There have been times when I've purposely and actively avoided seeing people and you know what, they were some of the most miserable times of my life. Maybe you don't even want to tell God how you feel and how you wish to have a family. Well, he already knows our thoughts and desires and we can always trust him.

Elisha, after discussion with his servant recognises the elephant in the room which is the couple's infertility and the woman's reluctance to discuss it or ask him for a family so he dives straight in,

'About this time next year,' Elisha said, 'you will hold a son in your arms.' 'No, my lord!' she objected. 'Please, man of God, don't mislead your servant!' But the woman became pregnant, and the next year about that same time she gave birth to a son, just as Elisha had told her.

(2 Kings 4:16–17)

This promise that Elisha gives the couple is similar to the one given by God to Abraham centuries earlier: 'Is anything too hard for the LORD? I will return to you at the appointed time next year, and Sarah will have a son' (Genesis 18:14). It's a great reminder of the consistent character of God through the Bible. Here He is years later doing the same miracles and he still wants to do those miracles today.

It's interesting that we don't really hear much about the husband in this story. You get the impression that the 'well-to-do' woman, the one who makes the decision to build a place for Elisha to stay at their home, is the dominant character, with her husband lurking in the background of the story. Elisha deals straight with the woman, asking her what he could do for her with no mention of her husband. In fact, the only thing we do know is that he is old – another common theme of the infertility stories of the Bible. When the child becomes unwell the husband appears to fail in his responsibilities as a caring father and sends the child to his mother. The husband wasn't even there when his son died and it was his wife who went to Elisha for help (2 Kings 4 v 18-22).

This example of a 'passive husband' really resonates with me. I'm pretty laid back and calm which is a good quality when dealing with medical emergencies at work but at home that can shift into me taking a back seat in our marriage and fail in my job as leader and husband. Too many times in our personal journey I've been found AWOL while Emma has been persistently pursuing God. Perhaps the Shunammite man had been close to giving up on God through years of disappointment, and his much longed for son's death was the final straw. We can all feel like giving up at times but the people who overcome are those who 'man up', keep on fighting (standing!), praying and trusting. The Shunammite man is not the image of husbands and fathers that God portrays in the Bible: Fathers who love no matter what their children do, as shown in the story of the prodigal son (Luke 15:11–32), who can't wait for their children to come home; God the Father, who continuously loves his children despite all their disobedience in the Old Testament, who declares:

'I have loved you with an everlasting love; I have drawn you with unfailing kindness' (Jeremiah 31:3).

Jesus is pictured as a loving husband who died for his bride, the church and this is the sacrificial love we should be demonstrating to our wives and families,

'Husbands, love your wives, just as Christ loved the church and gave himself up for her' (Ephesians 5:25).

Husbands and fathers should be lovingly leading their families and wives in their walk with God, willing to fight and die for them. Even though we may feel like giving up when we're disappointed, God hasn't and never will give up on us and so we should never give up on him or for caring for our wives either. The Shunammite woman certainly didn't give up even though her son had died and went to Elisha and insisted that he come to her son:

> When Elisha reached the house, there was the boy lying dead on his couch. He went in, shut the door on the two of them and prayed to the LORD. Then he got on the bed and lay on the boy, mouth to mouth, eyes to eyes, hands to hands. As he stretched himself out on him, the boy's body grew warm. Elisha turned away and walked back and forth in the room and then got on the bed and stretched out on him once more. The boy sneezed seven times and opened his eyes.
>
> Elisha summoned Gehazi and said, 'Call the Shunammite.' And he did. When she came, he said, 'Take your son.' She came in, fell at his feet and bowed to the ground. Then she took her son and went out.
>
> *(2 Kings 4:32–37)*

Because of her persistence the Shunammite woman received a healing resurrection for her son! How great an example to us of persevering even when things seem hopeless, not just with infertility but with our whole lives.

> Blessed is the one who perseveres under trial because, having stood the test, that person will receive the crown of life that the Lord has promised to those who love him.
>
> *(James 1:12)*

Lessons from the Shunammite man

- Don't be a passive husband or father.
- Don't give up on God.
- God is consistent in his miracles.

Discussion questions

- In which areas of my life am I not taking responsibility? Why?
- Am I good leader of my family? If not, why not?
- Am I persevering or ready to give up?

CHAPTER ELEVEN

Zechariah

Luke 1:5–80

I'm not sure about you but I find it really encouraging that right at the heart of the most significant story in history is a story of infertility (and adoption, but more on that later). When the world goes mad for tinsel, presents and Santa Claus, it is often forgotten that God places a couple who struggled to have children at the start of the Christmas story.

The birth of John the Baptist was prophesied through Malachi in chapter 3, verse 1: "'I will send my messenger, who will prepare the way before me. Then suddenly the Lord you are seeking will come to his temple; the messenger of the covenant, whom you desire, will come,' says the Lord Almighty.' Fast forward 400 years and this prophecy was still waiting to be fulfilled, the promised Messiah was still nowhere to be seen – it was beginning to look like God was never going to act (which is similar to that feeling of waiting in infertility). However, God was about to break His silence.

The story of Zechariah and Elizabeth is only found in the Gospel of Luke. I don't know why that is but I like to imagine that as a doctor Luke understood more than the other disciples how impossible this situation was and he found a medical miracle more remarkable than his fellow Gospel writers!

Zechariah, meaning 'God has remembered', was a priest and was married to Elizabeth, which means 'God's promise'. Both were descendants of Aaron the high priest, the brother of Moses. Luke 1:6 is one of the key verses in this story: 'Both of them were righteous in the sight of God, observing all the Lord's commands and decrees blamelessly.' Luke tells us they were both 'righteous' yet still they couldn't have children. It doesn't matter how good you are you can't do anything to be good enough to deserve children – they are a gift from a generous God. I know that I have fallen into that mindset of thinking I'm a 'good' Christian so I deserve for God to give me a child. Maybe Zechariah and Elizabeth felt the same? I guess we'll never know while we're on earth, but it's not impossible to imagine their disappointment and frustrations that after years of faithfully serving God they were still childless.

The painful truth is that none of us deserve anything from God and he has already given us his everything in Jesus. I wholeheartedly believe that infertility is not a punishment for past sins either. Whatever the Enemy tries to tell you, it's simply not true. God is still so gracious to us that he wants to bless us with good gifts, which I believe includes children, among other things.

We are told that Zachariah and Elizabeth were both very old and humanly speaking couldn't have children (Luke 1:7), but as we've already seen with Abraham and Sarah age is no barrier to God. While Zechariah is alone in the temple, an angel, who we later learn is Gabriel, appears to him and says: 'Do not be afraid, Zechariah; your prayer has been heard. Your wife Elizabeth will bear you a son, and you are to call him John' (Luke 1:13).

We don't know how long Zechariah and Elizabeth had been praying for a child, or even if their prayers had ceased. I have heard that a more accurate translation of verse 13 is the 'prayer you no longer pray has been heard' (emphasis mine). Even if we have lost hope and stopped praying, we can be assured that God has heard our prayers and they (and you) have not been forgotten. It says in 1 John 5: 14: 'This is the confidence we have in approaching God: that if we ask anything according to his will, he hears us.'

Gabriel tells Zechariah that he and Elizabeth will have a son and they are to call him John, meaning 'God is gracious'. You can picture Zechariah's shock and surprise at seeing an angel who then tells him he would be having a son – it's no wonder Gabriel said, 'Do not be afraid'! Gabriel goes on to tell Zechariah:

> He will be a joy and delight to you, and many will rejoice because of his birth, for he will be great in the sight of the Lord. He is never to take wine or other fermented drink, and he will be filled with the Holy Spirit even before he is born. He will bring back many of the people of Israel to the Lord their God. And he will go on before the Lord, in the spirit and power of Elijah, to turn the hearts of the parents to their children and the disobedient to the wisdom of the righteous – to make ready a people prepared for the Lord.
>
> *(Luke 1:14–17)*

When Zechariah hears this, he says, 'How can I be sure of this? I am an old man and my wife is well along in years' (Luke 1:18). Unlike Manoah in Judges 13, Zechariah doesn't quite have the faith to believe the words of Gabriel and so he asks for proof. He looks at his circumstances rather than to the One who has control of all circumstances.

I don't know what your infertility circumstances are. They may be old age, poor health, a low sperm count or something else. What I do know is that when faced with uncertainty we've got to focus on God for our source of confidence and strength. As it says in Joshua 1:9: 'Have I not commanded you? Be strong and courageous. Do not be afraid; do not be discouraged, for the Lord your God will be with you wherever you go.'

The angel continued speaking to Zechariah:

> I am Gabriel. I stand in the presence of God, and I have been sent to speak to you and to tell you this good news. And now you will be silent and not able to speak until the day this happens, because you did not believe my words, which will come true at their appointed time.
>
> *(Luke 1:19–20)*

So after Zechariah's doubt he ended up mute, but that didn't stop God from blessing them with a child. Even though we may struggle to have faith to believe a miracle is possible it won't stop God withholding blessings from us. I've heard it said that one of the reasons why God made Zechariah mute was to stop him speaking any more negative words and exclaiming his doubt. Even though God has promised us healing and wants to bless us we still need to be aware of the impact our words can have.

When the time comes for his son to be born, Zechariah shows his obedience to God's command:

> He asked for a writing tablet, and to everyone's astonishment he wrote, 'His name is John.' Immediately his mouth was opened and his tongue set free, and he began to speak, praising God. All the neighbours were filled with awe, and throughout the hill country of Judea people were

talking about all these things. Everyone who heard this wondered about it, asking, 'What then is this child going to be?' For the Lord's hand was with him.

(Luke 1:63–66)

The moment that Zechariah's speech was restored his first words were ones of praise to God! This should always be our response to God's goodness – gratitude and praise! It's always great to testify to other people about what God's done in your life; it can be a source of great encouragement to them and is, in fact, one of the main reasons that I wanted to write this book. No doubt, as prominent members of society, people may have gossiped about Zechariah and Elizabeth, particularly as the years went by and they remained childless, not least because it was believed at that time that sickness was the result of sin (see John 9:2). Those same people who may have been gossiping were now witnessing the miracle God had done in Zechariah and Elizabeth's lives – that's the life-changing power of testimony!

Seeing God at work is also incredibly encouraging and fills us with faith and confidence in what God can do. Luke 1:67 tells us that 'Zechariah was filled with the Holy Spirit' and went on to prophesy over his new son, echoing the words of Malachi: 'And you, my child, will be called a prophet of the Most High; for you will go on before the Lord to prepare the way for him' (Luke 1:76).

Zechariah had gone from a frightened, old, childless priest in verse 12 to a man filled with the Holy Spirit who understands God's plan for the salvation of mankind and the role his son will play in preparing the way for the coming Saviour. Our children also have great futures and roles to play for God in winning people back for him. We should embrace this and pray for their futures even though they may not yet be conceived. God has given me a Scripture for our children that I like to claim and prophesize over them: 'Very truly I tell you, whoever believes in me will do the works I have been doing, and they will do even greater things than these, because I am going to the Father' (John 14:12).

I pray that my children will be used mightily by God and do 'greater things than these'.

Lessons from Zechariah

- It doesn't matter how 'righteous' you are, you can't earn God's blessings.
- Our physical circumstances shouldn't dictate what God can do.
- We need to have faith that God will do what he promises.
- Give thanks to God for his blessings.
- Be aware of negative words.
- Testify to God's goodness.
- Prophesy for your children.

Discussion questions

- Have I given up praying or consistently praying for children?
- Do I feel a sense of entitlement from God for a family?
- In the things I do, am I trying 'to earn' a family from God?

CHAPTER TWELVE

The Men with No Children

There are people in the Bible who didn't have children just as not everyone was healed the most famous being Paul and his 'thorn' in his flesh (2 Corinthians 12 v 7) or Trophimus (2 Timothy 4 v 20). I want to be truthful and not shy away from this fact so we will look at these examples from Scripture.

Michal was the younger daughter of Saul, the first king of Israel. She was given in marriage to David after he presented her father with two hundred Philistine foreskins as told in 1 Samuel 18:20–27. When David was forced into exile she was given in marriage to another man, Paltiel son of Laish (1 Samuel 25:44). When David returned from exile as King of Judah he demanded that Saul's son Ish-Bosheth, who was king of Israel at that time, return Michal to him (2 Samuel 3:12–16). When Ish-Bosheth was killed David became king over the unified kingdom and brought the Ark of the Covenant to Jerusalem. David danced with joy in front of the Ark but Michal despised him in her heart:

> When David returned home to bless his household, Michal daughter of Saul came out to meet him and said, 'How the king of Israel has distinguished himself today, going around half-naked in full view of the slave girls of his servants as any vulgar fellow would!'

David said to Michal, 'It was before the LORD, who chose me rather than your father or anyone from his house when he appointed me ruler over the LORD's people Israel – I will celebrate before the LORD. I will become even more undignified than this, and I will be humiliated in my own eyes. But by these slave girls you spoke of, I will be held in honour.'

And Michal daughter of Saul had no children to the day of her death.

(2 Samuel 6:20–23)

We're not told why Michal had no children. Maybe David didn't sleep with her again after this incident, maybe it was to prevent the seed of Saul and David mixing so Saul had no inheritance of the coming Messiah Jesus, or maybe she had some illness that prevented her from having children. The truth is we don't know.

On two more occasions Scripture mentions people not being able to have children, both in 1 Chronicles 2: 'The sons of Nadab: Seled and Appaim. Seled died without children' (verse 30) and 'The sons of Jada, Shammai's brother: Jether and Jonathan. Jether died without children' verse 32).

Now again, we don't know the exact circumstances behind why these men died without children. They could have been unmarried or died young, or maybe they were unable to have them. We need to be very careful how we read and interpret Scripture. Theologian Dr. Donald A. Carson attributes his father as saying "a text taken out of context is a pretext for a proof text." meaning without examining the context in which scripture was said, you can easily (or even intentionally) misuse a text to support a position that it in fact does not support. However, I think it is significant that this has been included in Scripture and we know that 'All Scripture is God-breathed and is useful for teaching, rebuking, correcting and training in righteousness' (2 Timothy 3:16).

Even these lists of genealogies that we so often skip through can teach us something significant about our walk with Jesus. I don't believe that God would want anyone to not have children because of sickness and infertility but we live in a fallen world, a world that seems increasingly godless. Even though we live in difficult times now, in heaven there will be no more sickness or death. Jesus told us to pray, 'your kingdom come, your will be done, on earth as it is in heaven' (Matthew 6:10).

I don't want the fact that some people in the Bible may not have had children to set a precedent that we accept as normal today. As we have seen, God is consistent in his love, blessings and miracles. I want to see heaven on earth now, and part of that will be no more infertility. If Jesus told us to pray for heaven on earth we should pray for that and wait expectantly to see God at work.

Lessons from the Men with No children

- Be careful how we read and interpret scripture
- Don't skip through parts of the Bible we may think are insignificant

Discussion Questions

- How am I seeking heaven on earth?
- How do I read the Bible? What's my attitude?

PART THREE

Adoptions in the Bible

The first time I watched Disney's *The Jungle Book* as an adult I was with my daughter and I just couldn't stop crying! When my wife came into the room she thought something serious was wrong – it was pretty embarrassing! The part of the film that got me was at the beginning when the wolf family who 'adopt' Mowgli are told they need to take him back to the 'Man village'. Shere Khan, the tiger who 'hates man' (just like our Enemy), had returned to the jungle and was looking to kill Mowgli. Rama the wolf father says, 'The man-cub is like my own son. Surely he's entitled to the protection of the pack.'

Even though Mowgli wasn't his birth child (or more accurately birth wolf-cub!), Rama was still willing to protect him even if that meant putting his own life in danger. That captures perfectly the heart of how adopted parents feel about their children and how I felt about my daughter.

Adoption is not God's Plan B as we shall see in this final part. God the Father is the ultimate adopter, as Psalm 68 declares:

> A father to the fatherless, a defender of widows,
> is God in his holy dwelling.
> God sets the lonely in families ...
> *(Psalm 68:5–6)*

Whilst I was waiting to adopt I found it really encouraging to study the stories of adoption in the Bible and see how God uses those individuals to accomplish his purposes. It's great to see what lessons we can learn from the Bible – key principles that we can use in our own lives now and then as we parent children, whether birth or adopted. If you are still in the 'waiting' phase of your life I hope these stories will give you some food for thought about adoption and how you may parent in the future.

CHAPTER THIRTEEN

Moses

The story of Moses and his adoption by Pharaoh's daughter is remarkable and probably the most famous adoption story in all the Bible. Moses was the most significant man in the Old Testament, who God used to rescue the Israelites out of Egypt and brought the law to his people. The circumstances of his birth and adoption take place in Egypt where the Israelites, after settling in Egypt as a family of 70 (Jacob, his 12 sons and their families) had grown dramatically in number and had been put into slavery by Pharaoh to try to control their size. God knew how difficult this was going to be for his people and had planned for Moses to rescue them. Pharaoh recognized the threat the Israelites were to his kingdom,

> 'Look,' he said to his people, 'the Israelites have become far too numerous for us. Come, we must deal shrewdly with them or they will become even more numerous and, if war breaks out, will join our enemies, fight against us and leave the country.'
>
> *(Exodus 1:9–10)*

His plan was for the midwives to kill any male babies born to Israelite mothers. This scheme was unsuccessful because the midwives feared God more than Pharaoh and they let the

Israelite boys live. Pharaoh's next step was to declare, 'Every Hebrew boy that is born you must throw into the Nile, but let every girl live' (Exodus 1:22).

This is the situation that Moses' parents found themselves in. Amran, his father, and Jochebed, his mother, were both descended from the tribe of Levi. Can you envisage living in a time when the ruler of the land commands that you have to throw your baby son into a crocodile infested river? You couldn't think of anything worse. Interestingly, Mary and Joseph faced the same dilemma when King Herod ordered the massacre of all the baby boys at the time of Jesus' birth, but they escaped *to* Egypt. Moses' parents recognised he was no ordinary child and their faith in defying Pharaoh and trusting God was acknowledged in the book of Hebrews: 'By faith Moses' parents hid him for three months after he was born, because they saw he was no ordinary child, and they were not afraid of the king's edict' (Hebrews 11:23).

When Moses' parents could no longer hide him, his mother made a basket of papyrus reeds and placed him in the river Nile, instructing Moses' older sister Miriam to keep watch over him.

> Then Pharaoh's daughter went down to the Nile to bathe, and her attendants were walking along the riverbank. She saw the basket among the reeds and sent her female slave to get it. She opened it and saw the baby. He was crying, and she felt sorry for him. 'This is one of the Hebrew babies,' she said.
>
> Then his sister asked Pharaoh's daughter, 'Shall I go and get one of the Hebrew women to nurse the baby for you?'
>
> 'Yes, go,' she answered. So the girl went and got the baby's mother. Pharaoh's daughter said to her, 'Take this baby and nurse him for me, and I will pay you.' So the woman took

the baby and nursed him. When the child grew older, she took him to Pharaoh's daughter and he became her son. She named him Moses, saying, 'I drew him out of the water.'

(Exodus 2:5–10)

This Egyptian princess, whose name is unknown, is in some ways like Mary the mother of Jesus. Just as he does with Mary and Jesus, God entrusts a young woman to bring up a special child at potential great risk to herself. Mary suffered the shame of being seen to be the mother of an illegitimate child in an ultra conservative Jewish society, while Pharoah's daughter risked the wrath of her father by bringing a Hebrew child that he'd wanted dead into the royal household. Why Pharoah's daughter chose to do this we'll never know but her compassion and bravery in saving Moses' life was instrumental in God's plan to free his people from slavery and lead them on their journey to the Promised Land.

Moses certainly had a very interesting and significant childhood and education. Steven, the first Christian martyr, speaking centuries later during his trial gives this account of the first 40 years of Moses life, said:

As the time drew near for God to fulfil his promise to Abraham, the number of our people in Egypt had greatly increased. Then 'a new king, to whom Joseph meant nothing, came to power in Egypt.' He dealt treacherously with our people and oppressed our ancestors by forcing them to throw out their new born babies so that they would die.

At that time Moses was born, and he was no ordinary child. For three months he was cared for by his family. When he was placed outside, Pharaoh's daughter took him and brought him up as her own son. Moses was educated

in all the wisdom of the Egyptians and was powerful in
speech and action.

(Acts 7:17–22)

We've seen twice in Scripture Moses referred to as 'no ordinary
child'. I don't believe that there exists an *ordinary* child –
every child is a unique and special gift from God. As parents
one of our jobs is to find that God-given specialness in our
children and nurture that. There certainly was something
special about Moses that his parents instantly recognised and it
gave them courage to defy Pharaoh and allowed him to survive
to be the man who led his people to freedom.

Moses was brought up as a prince in the Egyptian royal
family. He must have had a life of extraordinary privilege – the
finest education, foods, beautiful clothes and slaves to meet his
every need. God knew that it would be necessary for Moses
to be brought up as a prince and not in slavery so he would
have the mindset of a prince and not of a pauper and slave.
His education would have included military studies of how to
lead an army and the tactics to fight battles. These were the
foundations for Moses to be able to lead the Israelites out of
Egypt, win wars against the surrounding peoples and write the
first five books of the Bible. Despite all the material delights
of Egypt Moses remained true to the faith of his birth, and
despite all this privilege he was willing to give it all up for God.
He could have had a life of comfort, chilling in the palace but
he chose not to:

By faith Moses, when he had grown up, refused to be
known as the son of Pharaoh's daughter. He chose to
be mistreated along with the people of God rather than
to enjoy the fleeting pleasures of sin. He regarded disgrace
for the sake of Christ as of greater value than the treasures

of Egypt, because he was looking ahead to his reward. By faith he left Egypt, not fearing the king's anger; he persevered because he saw him who is invisible.

(Hebrews 11:24-27)

What an incredible thing to have said about you – something we should aspire to. Moses ignored his circumstances and looked ahead to God, the plans for his life and his ultimate reward. A great example to us all no matter what our journey may hold.

From the life of Moses we see how God can use adoption for his divine purposes and that even though circumstances seem impossible God can make all things good. The decision to have children through adoption may have been made after years of frustrating infertility for some people. For Emma and I, when we think of our children now and how much we both love them, if God offered us the choice of them or 'birth' children we'd choose them every time! That's because we know and love them and we know how different their lives would have been if they hadn't been adopted. I believe the unique upbringing they'll have with us, just like the unique upbringing of Moses, will equip them with the skills and abilities to be used mightily by God. In the same way, being adopted into God's family for all believers means the difference between heaven and an eternity without God.

Moses faced many difficulties in his life. He was a prince of Egypt but he was born into a Hebrew slave family. He was aware of his heritage and in the book of Exodus, which most scholars presume to be written by Moses, he refers to the Israelites as 'his own people' (Exodus 2 v 11). It's important that while we bring our adoptive children up as our own flesh and blood that they also know the truth of their birth in an age appropriate way. We should always speak well and truthfully of their birth parents and not be afraid that they may prefer to be in their birth families. Children are naturally inquisitive and will want to know the truth about their families. Telling them the truth in an appropriate way will prevent them becoming confused and seeking to find answers in ways that might not be helpful, such as trying to find their family members on social media.

Exodus tells us that Moses had two older birth siblings, Miriam and Aaron, who played important roles in his life. We don't know anything about their relationships while Moses was a young boy and growing up as an Egyptian prince, but in later life they worked together to help bring the Israelites out of captivity. We read that Miriam watched over her helpless baby brother as he sailed down the Nile towards Pharaoh's daughter and then told the Egyptian princess that her mother could nurse the baby. Later, Miriam led the Israelites in worship after crossing the Red Sea and was called a prophetess. Aaron accompanied and supported his sibling when they went before Pharaoh to request that he let the Israelites leave Egypt. He also physically supported his brother by helping Moses hold up his staff in a battle against the Amalekites (Exodus 17) and helped lead the people through the wilderness. What a blessing it is to have family members to do life with and serve God alongside.

Although Moses' adoption was unique and nothing like the typical adoptions of our time, we can still learn important life lessons from it. Just as Moses, Miriam and Aaron shared the same family background, adopted children will always have a special bond with their birth siblings even if they haven't grown up together. Adopted children may be curious to know about and eventually meet any birth siblings and as adoptive parents we need to try to understand and respect this. We shouldn't be fearful about them meeting if an appropriate situation arises as this could be of tremendous benefit to them, and we know God can use all these situations and circumstances for his glory.

No relationships between siblings are perfect and this was true of Moses, Miriam and Aaron when they clashed over Moses' Cushite wife (Numbers 12) and there was jealousy that Moses was the sole leader. I'm sometimes guilty of unrealistic expectations and one of those was that our children would always get on perfectly! I don't think any siblings get on all the time and neither will yours (or ours!). Disagreements and squabbles are all part of learning and growing up and as parents we need to teach our children with love and grace how to interact with one another.

Due to his unusual upbringing, I wouldn't be surprised if Moses was sometimes confused about his true identity. The same may also be true of adopted children too who may have lived with different families over tiem. Eventually though, Moses did come to know his true identity; he wasn't an Egyptian prince, he wasn't a Levite, he wasn't a magician or miracle worker, he wasn't a man fearful of speaking in public, he wasn't a murderer, he wasn't a shepherd or leader of Israel. We are told, 'The LORD would speak to Moses face to face, as one speaks to a friend' (Exodus 33:11). It also says in Deuteronomy 34:10–12:

> Since then, no prophet has risen in Israel like Moses, whom the Lord knew face to face, who did all those signs and wonders the Lord sent him to do in Egypt – to Pharaoh and to all his officials and to his whole land. For no one has ever shown the mighty power or performed the awesome deeds that Moses did in the sight of all Israel.

His true identity was as God's friend, someone who had a face to face relationship with God! This incredible gift of friendship is available to us today too. Friendship with God is something that we should all be actively pursuing, and teaching our children to seek too. Nothing is more important than this relationship. Jesus said: 'I no longer call you servants, because a servant does not know his master's business. Instead, I have called you friends, for everything that I learned from my Father I have made known to you' (John 15:15).

If you ever have doubts that God wants to be friends with you and that you are adopted into his family, look what price he paid to make that friendship a reality – the blood of Jesus. Regardless of how our children come into our families this is the key thing we need to teach them: their foremost identity is that they are a child of God's and he wants to be friends with them.

Lessons from Moses

- God can turn difficult situations into opportunities to bless us.
- God keeps his promises.
- God uses adoption as part of his plans and purposes.
- Our identity is as a friend of God.
- Moses chose God over a lifetime of comfort.

Discussion questions

- As parents how much do we trust God with our children's lives?
- What are the similarities between the birth and adoptions of Jesus and Moses?
- What unique opportunities can I give to my children to prepare them for adult life?

- Do we struggle with our identities? How?
- What steps can I take to ensure our children, both birth and adopted, know their true identity?
- Do I know that I am adopted into God's family? If not, why not?
- Is God calling me to adopt?

CHAPTER FOURTEEN

Esther

Just like Moses, the story of Esther is another example of God using adoption in his purposes and plans to bring about the deliverance of his people.

To set the scene, as a result of years of disobedience and evil kings, the Jews had been taken into captivity in Babylon. As God had declared through Isaiah (44:28; 45:1) and Jeremiah (29:10), he hadn't forgotten them and had promised to bring them home; the captivity was coming to an end. In 537 BC a decree was issued by Cyrus the King of Persia (as predicted in Isaiah one hundred and fifty years before) where the Jews were allowed to return to Jerusalem. Some 50,000 Jews decided to make the long journey back to their home land to rebuild the temple. The story of Esther starts in 483 BC, between this first return of the Jewish exiles and the second return led by Ezra the priest in 458 BC.

Esther was a Jew who was adopted by her cousin Mordecai after her parents died (Esther 2 v 7). Mordecai, like Boaz in the story of Ruth, was a 'kinsman redeemer'. A kinsman redeemer was the nearest male relative who had the responsibility to help a relative who was in trouble or danger. It is again a picture of Jesus who redeems us. It would be unusual in today's times for both parents to die and for a child to be brought up by a relative but it does still happen. Sometimes family members for whatever reasons are not able to look after their children and so they are brought up by their extended family. Maybe this is a situation you find yourself in now.

Xerxes I was the king of Persia and the ruler of the largest empire the world had ever seen. It covered the area now known as Turkey, Iraq, Iran, Pakistan, Jordan, Lebanon, Israel and sections of modern-day Egypt, Sudan, Libya and Saudi Arabia. At that time he was the most powerful man on earth and yet God used an apparently insignificant girl, an orphan amongst a captive nation to marry the king and save His people again!

Xerxes began searching for another wife after being publicly humiliated by his wife Queen Vashti. Esther was amongst the girls chosen as a possible new wife. God was with Esther and we are told on three occasions that she won favour with different people (Esther 2:9, 15, 17). Esther was taken to live in the royal palace and put through a year-long beauty regime (Esther 2 v 12) before she was then taken to Xerxes. He was so delighted with her that she was chosen to become queen.

Soon after Esther became queen, an official named Haman was brought to prominence in the kingdom and honoured by King Xerxes. Haman was a descendent of Agag, king of the Amalekites who were long-time enemies of the Jewish people. Esther's uncle Mordecai often came into contact with Haman but refused to bow to him because as a Jew he would only bow to God. Haman hated Mordecai for this and with King Xerxes' permission plotted to kill all the Jews in the country. When this genocidal edict is announced Mordecai sends a message to Esther warning her about what was being planned and how it would lead to her death too:

Do not think that because you are in the king's house you alone of all the Jews will escape. For if you remain silent at this time, relief and deliverance for the Jews will arise from another place, but you and your father's family will perish. And who knows but that you have come to your royal position for such a time as this?

(Esther 4:13–14)

You may not be a queen (or king!), but God can use you 'for such a time as this'. It may be through a challenging circumstance or situation that God presents you with an opportunity to stand up for him, witness to a colleague or pray for someone's healing. The problem with opportunities is that they may be unique and only come around once in a lifetime. When we stepped into our adoption journey, we felt this was our 'for such a time as this' moment. We get the privilege of sharing our faith with our children and like Mordecai we can bring our children up to be world changers too.

Thankfully, Esther was willing to risk her life for her people and tells Mordecai: 'Go, gather together all the Jews who are in Susa, and fast for me. Do not eat or drink for three days, night or day. I and my attendants will fast as you do. When this is done, I will go to the king, even though it is against the law. And if I perish, I perish' (Esther 4:16).

God granted Esther success and the king received her. Due to Esther's courage Haman's plot was exposed, the Jews were saved and Mordecai was promoted to second in charge in the country. Moredecai clearly took his parental responsibilities to Esther very seriously. Whilst she was preparing to meet the king we are told that he visited her everyday (Esther 2 v 11) and it is his wise counsel that guides her into saving the Jews. Parenthood is a sacred responsibility that we need to take seriously. Who knows what amazing things our children will accomplish with our love and guidance!

Lessons from Esther

- God will always find a way to save his people.
- We must be willing to make sacrifices for God.
- God can use the seemingly insignificant to influence the most important people in society.
- Mordecai took his parental responsibilities extremely seriously

Discussion questions

- Am I willing to sacrifice my own dreams, lifestyle or even life for God?
- Is there a 'for such a time as now' moment in my life where I have a unique opportunity? What do I need to do about it?
- Is fear holding me back in any areas of my life?
- Am I or how can I in the future bring my children up to be world changers?

CHAPTER FIFTEEN

Jesus

The most significant man who ever lived, the Son of God himself, was raised as an adopted child. Just let that sentence sink in. Read it again. I've been in church my entire life but never really noticed this significant fact or heard it preached on. God's own Son was in a sense *adopted* by Joseph, his earthly father.

Just like Moses, Jesus was born at a time when an evil, tyrannical king, who called himself Herod the Great, felt threatened and ordered that all the baby boys under two years old were to be killed: 'When Herod realised that he had been outwitted by the Magi, he was furious, and he gave orders to kill all the boys in Bethlehem and its vicinity who were two years old and under, in accordance with the time he had learned from the Magi' (Matthew 2:16).

The similarities between the life of Moses and Jesus are striking. Both were adopted as babies, brought up by birth mothers, rejected by the people they came to save, were shepherds and prophets, etc. This is an example of 'typology' in Scripture, where a person or thing in the Old Testament foreshadows a person or thing in the New Testament. It also fulfilled a prophecy made by Moses himself about the coming Messiah: 'The LORD your God will raise up for you a prophet like me from among you, from your fellow Israelites. You must listen to him' (Deuteronomy 18:15).

Joseph (meaning 'he will add or increase') was the man chosen by God to be the 'adoptive' father of Jesus. It's crazy to see in the genealogies (Matthew 1:1–17; Luke 3:23–38) that Jesus, through his adopted father Joseph and birth mother Mary, was a direct descendant of King David and Abraham! Genealogies were very important to the Jews and Jesus' family line going all the way back to Adam proves his identity as the Messiah by fulfilling Old Testament prophecies. Knowing our family backgrounds is important to us too and will be for adopted children when they are old enough to understand their past. Included in Jesus' genealogy were murderers, liars, adulterers and prostitutes; the Bible doesn't shy away from this. It's possible our adopted children will have relatives with difficult backgrounds. We have to be sensitive to this and help them understand that whatever is in our past is simply that – past. Our future is for us to decide and we can choose Jesus to lead us for the best future possible.

For me, Joseph is a remarkable man who doesn't get the credit he deserves for what he did in Jesus' early life. It's quite easy to gloss over his role in the Christmas story but what he did deserves a lot of respect. Joseph was already engaged to Mary when he found out that she was pregnant. Quite understandably, at first he didn't believe her story about being pregnant by the power of God, but because he was a 'righteous' man he planned to divorce her quietly even though by Jewish law Mary could have been stoned to death! It's then that God intervenes and sends the angel Gabriel to speak to Joseph through a dream:

'Joseph son of David, do not be afraid to take Mary home as your wife, because what is conceived in her is from the Holy Spirit. She will give birth to a son, and you are to give him the name Jesus, because he will save his people from their sins.'

All this took place to fulfil what the Lord had said through the prophet: 'The virgin will conceive and give birth to a son, and they will call him Immanuel' (which means 'God with us').

When Joseph woke up, he did what the angel of the Lord had commanded him and took Mary home as his wife. But he did not consummate their marriage until she gave birth to a son. And he gave him the name Jesus.

(Matthew 1:20–25)

Joseph initially had serious doubts about marrying Mary and taking on a son who wasn't his birth child. A 'cheating' wife and illegitimate son would have brought great shame on his family and ruined his reputation. It's no wonder that Joseph was planning to privately divorce Mary and abandon her unborn baby. To say that Joseph was a reluctant adopter is an understatement as it would have cost Joseph a lot to trust God's word to him. Fortunately for us, we see that Joseph was obedient to God in marrying Mary and being Jesus' earthly father. Obviously your own unique situation will be different to that faced by Joseph. Maybe your wife (or future wife) has children from a previous relationship and you're scared and having doubts about taking on and 'adopting' her children. It may be that pursuing adoption is what God has quietly been speaking to you about but you're afraid just like Joseph was. I ashamedly admit that I was a slightly reluctant adopter. You have fears that the children won't look like you, won't like the same sports or hobbies as you or reject you when they get older for not being their 'real dad'. I've got news for you: birth children could do all these things as well! That's the risk you take as a parent whichever way your children come along and we have to pray regularly for them while also giving them the freedom to make their own in choices in life. You may also worry what your parents or in-laws will think. Will they love the adopted children as much as birth children or will they reject them? I'm pleased to say that both sets of grandparents in our family would not consider for one second that our adopted children are inferior to any other grandchildren. All I can say is that adopting has been the best decision we have ever made as a couple. It's certainly not easy, but we've never regretted it and I'm sure Joseph didn't regret it either! Although adoption may not be right for everyone, if God is putting those desires in you and your wife's heart you need to be obedient to him and explore the possibilities of adoption yourselves.

Even though God had spoken to Joseph through a dream, I expect there were times when Joseph doubted the truth of the situation and questioned whether Mary may have been unfaithful. For the duration of his life Joseph would have been the subject of gossip that Jesus was illegitimate and not really his son. Maybe you are worried about others' opinions or if people are gossiping about you and your family too. It's not right and it can hurt, but adopted children are just as much part of God's plan for families as birth children. You can't argue with that because God chose that for his own Son!

Joseph recognised the responsibility he had as Jesus' father. Gabriel had revealed that Jesus was the child prophesied in Isaiah 7 v 14, the Son of God who was going to save his people. We as parents or parents to be, whilst maybe not having the same level of responsibility as Joseph had with Jesus, do still have a huge responsibility bringing up our own children. We need to ask God for his plans and purposes for their lives, to help us look for their gifts and skills, so that we can develop and encourage them to become all that God has created them to be.

We know Joseph was a carpenter and that he passed this skill onto Jesus (Mark 6 v 3). You can visualise the two of them side by side, the hours that they would have spent together, the father teaching his son the skills required for the trade. The most important thing we can give our children is quality time and so, just as Joseph invested his time into Jesus, we need to invest our time into our children too. It's so easy to become distracted by our phones, TV or simply just needing time alone to switch off when we are at home, but nothing is more important than the time we give to our children. I'm as guilty of this as anyone and one of the worst moments of my parenting life was when my oldest daughter became distraught when I answered a text message while she was telling me about her day at school. We mustn't see our children as an inconvenience when we get tired or busy. We need to make the conscious decision daily to give them the best of us. Seth and Lauren Dahl in their book Win+Win Parenting put it like this:

> Valuing our children and where they are on their journey through life is a choice. It's a wake up every morning and say, 'It won't be like this for long, I'm going to enjoy it and get absolutely every wonderful thing out of it I possibly can,' kind of choice. It's deliberate and intentional.

Giving quality time and being fully switched on with our children gives them a solid, loving foundation, creates lifelong bonds and helps them develop the godly character they will need in later life.

The last time we hear of Joseph is the story of a 12-year-old Jesus getting lost in Jerusalem during the Passover Festival (Luke 2:41–51). Can you imagine the terror of losing your child for three days? Can you then multiply that and think what losing the Son of God would feel like! That must have been the most incredibly stressful three days of searching ever! When Jesus' parents finally found him in the temple, Mary and Joseph failed to understand what he meant and why he was there:

> After three days they found him in the temple courts, sitting among the teachers, listening to them and asking them questions. Everyone who heard him was amazed at his understanding and his answers. When his parents saw him, they were astonished. His mother said to him, 'Son, why have you treated us like this? Your father and I have been anxiously searching for you.'
>
> 'Why were you searching for me?' he asked. 'Didn't you know I had to be in my Father's house?' But they did not understand what he was saying to them.
>
> *(Luke 2:46–50)*

As we discussed with Moses, adopted children may struggle with their identity. Jesus, as in all ways, is the perfect example of an adopted child – he knew who his true father was as evidenced by his reply to his parents when they found him, but he still loved and respected his earthly parents. We need to ensure our children, whether birth or adopted, know who their true heavenly Father is. This is my prayer for our children; that they know their identity as a child of God but also know and respect me as their earthly father.

At the conclusion of the story of Jesus getting lost in Jerusalem we are told that he 'went down to Nazareth with them and was obedient to them. But his mother treasured all these things in her heart. And Jesus grew in wisdom and stature, and in favour with God and man (Luke 2:51–52). It's important we demonstrate these principles to our children and explain that even Jesus was obedient to his earthly parents!

Lessons from Jesus

- God can speak to us clearly through dreams.
- God consistently makes bad situations into good.
- Obedience leads to blessings.

Discussion questions

- How was Jesus the perfect child?
- Do I know God as my heavenly father?
- Am I spending enough time with my children? If not, how can I plan to improve this?
- What am I teaching my children through my actions and words?
- Is God asking me to consider adoption?

CHAPTER SIXTEEN

Genubath

1 Kings 11:19–20

I hadn't heard of Genubath and I'll bet not many other people know this story! This is a very short passage which tells us about a man named Genubath, a man who was adopted by an Egyptian pharaoh's wife. We follow a God who hides gold and diamonds deep down in rocks for us to find and so we must dig deep for the treasure that's hidden in Scripture. As it says in Proverbs, 'It is the glory of God to conceal a matter; to search out a matter is the glory of kings' (Proverbs 25:2). There is 'treasure' hidden all through the Bible if we will search for it.

The origins of this story are found with King David's son Solomon. When Solomon became king he asked God for wisdom (1 Kings 3 v 3-15) and became known all around the world for his wisdom. Sadly, he was also known for the number of wives he had (1,000 – imagine that!) and this was ultimately the source of his downfall as his wives led him to worship idols. Because Solomon followed his wives in worshipping foreign idols God said he would take Solomon's kingdom away.

Another way that trouble came to Solomon was through Hadad, from the royal family of Edom. The Edomites had been almost completely destroyed by Israel. Hadad was only a child at that time and escaped to Egypt where the pharaoh provided for him. We are told:

> Pharaoh was so pleased with Hadad that he gave him a sister of his own wife, Queen Tahpenes, in marriage. The sister of Tahpenes bore him a son named Genubath, whom Tahpenes brought up in the royal palace. There Genubath lived with Pharaoh's own children.
>
> *(1 Kings 11:19–20)*

It appears from these two verses that Genubath was adopted into the royal family. It's difficult to make too much from such a short story, and we must exercise caution, but we do have authority to use *all* Scripture for learning and no piece of Scripture is insignificant. Here we have the picture of a child adopted into a royal family just as we are adopted into God's eternal royal family when we become his followers. That picture of undeserved grace is so powerful, even now thousands of years later. Presumably Genubath would have had the same privileges that the other Egyptian princes had, and indeed we have the same privileges and inheritance Jesus has as the Son of God now that we are adopted into God's family.

Lessons from Genubath

- No matter how wise we are, our lives can come to disaster if we take our focus off God.
- An insignificant individual was adopted into a royal family, just as we are adopted into God's eternal royal family.
- We can learn so much from studying the details of Scripture.

Discussion questions

- What treasures in Scripture am I missing?
- How can I find all the treasures hidden in Scripture?
- Do I trust in God or my own wisdom and intellect like Solomon?

CHAPTER SEVENTEEN

Naomi

The story of Naomi, whose name means 'sweat and pleasant', is found in the book of Ruth. Naomi, along with her husband and two sons, moves from Bethlehem to Moab to escape a famine in Judea. Her sons marry Moabite women Orpah and Ruth. When her husband and sons die Naomi and Ruth return to Bethlehem. Ruth ends up marrying a man named Boaz and gives birth to a son called Obed.

> Then Naomi took the child in her arms and cared for him. The women living there said, 'Naomi has a son!' And they named him Obed. He was the father of Jesse, the father of David.
>
> *(Ruth 4:16–17)*

The Hebrew word *aman* that was translated as 'cared for' in the NIV can have several meanings and so other versions of the Bible translate verse 16 slightly differently: 'Naomi took the baby and cuddled him to her breast. And she cared for him as if he were her own' (New Living Translation); 'And Naomi took the child, and laid it in her bosom, and became nurse unto it' (King James Version).

We can't know for sure whether Naomi actually breastfed Obed. Naomi herself said she was too old to have a husband

(Ruth 1:12) but if she managed to breastfeed Obed at an advanced age it would be no greater a miracle than that of Sarah having a child aged 90, or indeed any of the other miracles in the Bible! It may just be figurative speech for spiritual nourishment that a grandparent can give to a long hoped for grandchild.

Both Obed's parents, Boaz and Ruth, were alive at the time of his birth so Naomi didn't adopt him as a parent per se, but in a sense he would have felt like a son to her because he replaced her sons who had died, and doubtless she would have had a great influence on his life. Obed was another significant man who grew up to be the father of Jesse and hence was the grandfather of King David and therefore a direct ancestor of Jesus.

CHAPTER EIGHTEEN

Solomon and the Prostitutes

1 Kings 3:16–28

At first glance this story doesn't appear to have much to do with adoption but on closer study I think it does reveal an important truth about women who for whatever reason lose parental rights of their children or choose to give them up for adoption. The story of Solomon and the prostitutes is found in 1 Kings 3:16–28. Two prostitutes give birth to baby boys within three days of each other. The son of one of the women dies when she lies on him during the night so she exchanges the dead baby for the other woman's living son. The other woman recognises the deception and they go to Solomon to solve their dispute:

> The king said, 'This one says, "My son is alive and your son is dead," while that one says, "No! Your son is dead and mine is alive."'
>
> Then the king said, 'Bring me a sword.' So they brought a sword for the king. He then gave an order: 'Cut the living child in two and give half to one and half to the other.'
>
> The woman whose son was alive was deeply moved out of love for her son and said to the king, 'Please, my lord, give her the living baby! Don't kill him!'

But the other said, 'Neither I nor you shall have him. Cut him in two!'

Then the king gave his ruling: 'Give the living baby to the first woman. Do not kill him; she is his mother.'

(1 Kings 3:23–27)

The love of a mother for her child is an extraordinary thing! The Hebrew word *rahamim*, which is translated in this Scripture as 'deeply moved' (v 26), is related to *rehem*, meaning 'womb', and is especially appropriate for a mother's love. It mirrors the sacrificial love of God for his people. It reminds me of a tragic incident involving some of our friends and their children when we were working in Uganda. One night when the father was away their house caught fire and the mother kept running into her burning house to rescue her children. She managed to get them all out but tragically she died from smoke inhalation. Our friend made the ultimate sacrifice to save the lives of her children.

The mother of the living baby in the story was willing to sacrifice her own happiness to save her child from being killed, in effect allowing the other woman to adopt her child to prevent him from being killed. It's difficult to understand how hard it must be to give a child up for adoption or have a child taken away, but this is a common situation people all around the world find themselves in. Through ill health or difficult social circumstances parents may decide that their child will be better off being brought up by another family and that is an incredible sacrifice to make. No parent ever sets out to be a 'bad parent' and if they are struggling it is often because they are the victims of a troubled upbringing. We should always be empathetic towards adopted children's birth parents and consider their feelings and continue to pray for them.

I think it's interesting to note that Solomon makes no judgement or condemnation of the women's lifestyles and gives them the justice that they deserve. Our adopted children's birth parents may have made some bad choices in life (which we all can do from time to time) but they are still loved by God as much as you and me – Jesus still died for them – and so we need to remember them and pray that they will also find salvation.

Lessons from Solomon and the prostitutes

- Parents make sacrificial choices for their children.
- Don't judge other people.

Discussion questions

- If I have adopted children, do I pray for their birth parents? Why, or why not?
- What length would you go to protect any children you may have?

CHAPTER NINETEEN

Israel

God chose the nation of Israel as his own special possession and so adopted them as his children:

> For you are a people holy to the LORD your God. The LORD your God has chosen you out of all the peoples on the face of the earth to be his people, his treasured possession.
>
> The LORD did not set his affection on you and choose you because you were more numerous than other peoples, for you were the fewest of all peoples. But it was because the LORD loved you and kept the oath he swore to your ancestors that he brought you out with a mighty hand and redeemed you from the land of slavery, from the power of Pharaoh king of Egypt.
>
> *(Deuteronomy 7:6–8)*

Our adopted children haven't done anything to deserve our love. We have chosen them to be our children. We choose, just as God does, to love and shower our blessings on them.

In Hosea, God refers to the Israelites as his 'son': 'When Israel was a child, I loved him, and out of Egypt I called my son' (Hosea 11:1). (This verse is also described in Matthew as a prophetic picture of Jesus being called out of Egypt after Herod had died, see Matthew 2:13–15.)

In the same chapter of Hosea there is a beautiful picture of God, like a human father, describing how he taught his people and children (referred to as Ephraim, a tribe of Israel) to walk, how he leads them lovingly, how he bends down, picks them up and brings them close to his cheek to feed them:

It was I who taught Ephraim to walk,
    taking them by the arms;
but they did not realise
    it was I who healed them.
I led them with cords of human kindness,
    with ties of love.
To them I was like one who lifts
    a little child to the cheek,
    and I bent down to feed them.

(Hosea 11:3–4)

Not only is this showing how God led his people from slavery to the Promised Land but it shows us how we are to love and care for our children. It describes God as a human parent, caring for children as parents have done for thousands of years.

Jeremiah uses similar imagery when he describes how, like an earthly father, God supports his children: 'I will lead them beside streams of water on a level path where they will not stumble, because I am Israel's father, and Ephraim is my firstborn son' (Jeremiah 31:9).

Later in the same chapter, in his famous letter to the rebellious captives living in Babylon, Jeremiah is prophesying a time of restoration for God's people who had abandoned him: 'Is not Ephraim my dear son, the child in whom I delight? Though I often speak against him, I still remember him. Therefore my heart yearns for him; I have great compassion for him," declares the LORD' (Jeremiah 31:20).

Even though his children had rejected Him, God was still desperate for them to return to him. Despite this his people were still being disciplined for their sins as any good parent must discipline their children when they do wrong:

My son, do not despise the LORD's discipline,
    and do not resent his rebuke,
because the LORD disciplines those he loves,
    as a father the son he delights in.

(Proverbs 3:11–12)

God was still merciful to his children, always willing to forgive, just as we need to be with our children too. Children, whether adopted or not, need our discipline but they also need to know they are loved unconditionally, just as God loves us.

CHAPTER TWENTY

Adopted into God's Family

This last chapter could the most significant chapter in the book. We may be blessed with many children but, ultimately, if we haven't been adopted into God's family we miss the greatest blessing of all. As I've said previously, adoption is at the very heart of the Gospel. This form of adoption is not humans adopting other humans but God adopting us as his children to be part of his heavenly family. John puts it like this:

> Yet to all who did receive him, to those who believed in his name, he gave the right to become children of God – children born not of natural descent, nor of human decision or a husband's will, but born of God.
>
> *(John 1:12–13)*

In the New Testament, the Greek word for adoption is *huiothesia* and it is used on five occasions, three of those in Romans. It literally means 'to place as a son' and is defined in Louw and Nida's *Greek-English Lexicon* as this: 'to formally and legally declare that someone who is not one's own child is henceforth to be treated and cared for as one's own child, including complete rights of inheritance.'

The significance of Paul using this particular word to his Roman audience is very important. Unlike Jews, the Romans were very familiar with the process of adoption, where families would adopt healthy children, most often boys, to carry on the family name if their family had no birth children or only girls. According to Roman law, the adopted individual lost all rights to their old family and gained all the rights as a legitimate child of their new family. They became heir to their new family's possessions, legally their old life was wiped out including the cancellation of any debts and they became legally the son or daughter of their new parents.

From a Christian perspective you can see why salvation and adoption are so strongly linked and why Roman readers would understand completely the adoption references. As an adopted person in the first century AD your old life was finished, your debts were cancelled and you became a new person with a new family. It's a stunning picture of what happens at salvation where your sins are cancelled and you get a new heavenly family!

This is the first of Paul's references to adoption in the book of Romans: 'The Spirit you received does not make you slaves, so that you live in fear again; rather, the Spirit you received brought about your adoption to sonship. And by him we cry, "*Abba*, Father"' (Romans 8:15).

As sons and daughters of God we don't need to live in slavery to fear, or indeed to addiction, anger, doubt or any other sins that entangle and restrict our lives. Infertility may have enslaved your mind to the extent that you no longer trust God or have hope for a better future. Jesus wants to set you free right now from the prison that is in your mind. Incredibly, we have the joy and right to call God '*Abba*', an Aramaic word which translates as 'daddy', as a young child would call their father. This highlights the intimate, close father-child relationship God wishes for us all to have with him. No formalities, just an open, loving relationship.

Later in the same chapter Paul says: 'Not only so, but we ourselves, who have the first fruits of the Spirit, groan inwardly as we wait eagerly for our adoption to sonship, the redemption of our bodies' (Romans 8:23).

This verse reminds us that although we are part of God's family when we accept salvation, we are still yearning for that day when we finally go home to heaven and sin and sickness will be no more.

In Romans 9 Paul shows his love for his own people and desperation to win them for Christ:

> For I could wish that I myself were cursed and cut off from Christ for the sake of my people, those of my own race, the people of Israel. Theirs is the adoption to sonship; theirs the divine glory, the covenants, the receiving of the law, the temple worship and the promises.
>
> *(Romans 9:3–4)*

Paul also mentions adoption in two of his epistles. In his letter to the Galatians Paul summarises the Gospel like this:

> But when the set time had fully come, God sent his Son, born of a woman, born under the law, to redeem those under the law, that we might receive adoption to sonship. Because you are his sons, God sent the Spirit of his Son into our hearts, the Spirit who calls out, '*Abba*, Father.' So you are no longer a slave, but God's child; and since you are his child, God has made you also an heir.
>
> *(Galatians 4:4–7)*

In a Scripture that is quite similar to Romans 8:15, Paul is again equating salvation to being adopted into God's heavenly family. God had to redeem us as sons and daughters with the sacrifice of Jesus. That redemption was costly, and for adoptive parents adoption will be emotionally (and financially!) costly but that cost, as it is for God, is well worth it.

In Ephesians, Paul says that before God even created the world we had been chosen by him:

> For he chose us in him before the creation of the world to be holy and blameless in his sight. In love he predestined us for adoption to sonship through Jesus Christ, in accordance with his pleasure and will.
>
> *(Ephesians 1:4–5)*

No-one deserves to be saved, but God in his grace chose to save us! Whether we choose to accept this gift is up to us.

Conclusion

Through this book we've examined the stories in the Bible that deal with infertility and adoption. We've seen how God wants us to be fruitful, how he is our Healer and that he uses adoption to save his people and for the salvation of mankind. We've also read about how God is consistent in his nature and continues to bring hope, comfort and healing to men and their wives to overcome infertility today. Hopefully everything that you've read will help you 'man up' in a Godly way to be who you were created to be and not robbed by infertility.

Personally, I am trusting in God's kingdom plans for healing and believe it is still possible for my wife and I to have a birth child too. I am able to be joyful in God because he is my Saviour and that can never be taken away from me! The same principle can apply to any other areas of barrenness you may find in your life, be they financial, health, family or anything else. No matter what challenges we are facing, having God as our Saviour is a constant source of joy. Because I have been saved by God, I now understand more fully the joy of adoption and I'm so grateful that God has given me the privilege of being '*Abba*, father' to our children too. We are incredibly thankful for the blessing of children and for the joy and restoration their story brings.

I hope you are feeling encouraged to be an overcomer in whatever difficulties you are facing in your life today. God is the same yesterday, today and forever and wants to bless you abundantly in every area of your life.

My final question to you is this: will you trust him and be obedient to his plans and purposes for your life today?

The Science of Infertility

This part has purposely been put at the end, not because I want it to have the final word but because compared to God and his truth it's insignificant. It's not intended as medical advice – for that I'd encourage you to see your own doctor – but simply to give a basic understanding of the medical issues you or your wife may be facing.

The World Health Organisation defines infertility as 'a disease of the reproductive system defined by the failure to achieve a clinical pregnancy after 12 months or more of regular unprotected sexual intercourse.'

Basically, if you've not got pregnant within a year technically you're infertile. Infertility problems are increasing and more and more people are seeking medical advice for fertility problems. The medical facts of the matter are that most couples will conceive but that doesn't mean that it is always easy. Where the woman in under the age of 40, 80 per cent of couples will conceive within one year, rising to 90 per cent in two years.

The main causes of infertility in the UK are:

* problems with a woman's ovulation cycle (25%);
* damage to the ovarian tubes (20%);

- male problems causing infertility (30%);
- uterine (womb) or abdominal disorders (10%);
- unexplained infertility, meaning no obvious identified male or female cause (25%).

In about 40 per cent of cases, disorders are found in both the man and the woman. Uterine or endometrial factors, gamete or embryo defects, and pelvic conditions such as endometriosis may also play a role.

Once a diagnosis has been established, treatment falls into three main types:

- medical treatment to restore fertility, for example, the use of drugs such as Clomid to kick-start ovulation (egg production);
- surgical treatment to restore fertility, for example, removal of fibroids from the womb or burning off patches of endometriosis;
- assisted reproduction techniques (ART) – any treatment that deals with means of conception other than vaginal intercourse. It frequently involves the handling of gametes or embryos such as in in vitro fertilization (IVF).

I think we need to be wise and prayerful about using medication to help us get pregnant. In his book *Kisses from A Good God*, Paul Manwaring, a pastor at Bethel Church in California, says that 'medicine and surgery are not second-class healings'. I agree with this but they should never replace God as our hope for healing.

IVF, if it leads to destruction or freezing of embryos, can lead to difficult decisions for Christians who believe that life begins at fertilisation. It's costly from an emotional and financial point of view and success rates can vary widely. It's beyond the scope of this book to discuss these issues in any depth but we need to be aware of these issues and consider wisely.

What can I do as a man to improve my fertility?

I wouldn't be a good doctor if I didn't tell you to eat healthily, do plenty of exercise, watch your alcohol intake and stop smoking if you do – so consider yourself told!

Alcohol

Most men enjoy a beer (or two!). Excessive alcohol use can reduce testosterone levels and reduce sperm quality. The evidence suggests that three to four units per week is unlikely to affect your fertility but excessive alcohol can. If you're drinking heavily seek medical help to cut down.

Smoking

Smoking, and even passive smoking, has been shown to reduce fertility. If you do smoke get some help to stop – it's the worst thing you can do for your health!

Obesity

Having a Body Mass Index (BMI) over 30 for women can delay conception and cause ovulation problems. Obese men will also be less fertile.

Cycling

I've put this in for my wife because I love cycling and so she's got no excuse for telling me off for going cycling. Thankfully there's no evidence that suggests cycling affects a man's fertility!

Investigations for men

Semen is checked for the quantity and quality of sperm. Some men have a low sperm count or even no sperm in their semen at all, which can be caused by a blockage in the tubes that carry the sperm. If you are one of those men, you must not beat yourself up about it. You need to know your worth is not calculated by your sperm count (or your salary, house, car or whatever else the world counts as valuable); you're worth what God thinks you're worth and that price was his own Son's life.

Investigations for women

Hysterosalpingography (HSG)

Dye is inserted into the cervix which then spreads to the fallopian tubes. An X-ray is then taken to check that they are still open and will allow an egg to pass down them.

Chlamydia

Testing for the sexually transmitted disease chlamydia should be performed as symptoms can be minimal in women. This infection can cause pelvic inflammatory disease, which leads to infertility by scarring of the fallopian tubes, as well as increasing the risk of miscarriage and ectopic pregnancy (when a pregnancy develops outside of the womb, most commonly the fallopian tubes).

If you have any concerns about the above please make an appointment to see your GP.

The final word

I've talked a lot about Jesus in this book, how much He's done in my life and how he helps me everyday. I gave my life to

Jesus as a seven-year-old boy and it was the greatest decision I ever made. I want to take this opportunity to ask you to think about what you believe about Jesus. If you aren't a Christian but want to follow Jesus as your personal saviour this is what the Bible says,

If you declare with your mouth, "Jesus is Lord," and believe in your heart that God raised him from the dead, you will be saved. For it is with your heart that you believe and are justified, and it is with your mouth that you profess your faith and are saved. Romans 10 v 9-10

To start on this incredible journey and become God's 'adopted' child pray this prayer and ask Jesus into your life,

'Dear Lord Jesus, I know that I am a sinner, and I ask for Your forgiveness. I believe You died for my sins and rose from the dead. I turn from my sins and invite You to come into my heart and life. I want to trust and follow You as my Lord and Saviour.'

If you've prayed this prayer I'd love to hear from you so I can pray.

Blessings
Pete